Advance Praise for
Mind Over Menopause

"Menopause is more than hot flashes, vaginal dryness, or even deciding whether to use hormones. Leslee Kagan and Bruce Kessel have explored the many facets of this important transition for women. They have charted an approach that will help women to make the last third of their lives the best."

—Marcie Richardson, M.D., Codirector
of Harvard Vanguard Menopause Consultation Service

"At a time when hormone therapy has been called into question, three distinguished experts have shared their knowledge concerning nonhormonal treatment. Women entering the menopause need to know their options for relieving symptoms. This book is beautifully written. It will certainly become part of my library and a recommendation for my patients."

—Isaac Schiff, M.D., Professor and Chief
of the Obstetrics and Gynecology Service,
Massachusetts General Hospital

"Now that women are no longer taking hormone replacement therapy for menopausal symptoms, they need alternative remedies. The problems of menopause respond very well to mind/body interventions. This book gives you the practical advice you need to take advantage of the power of the mind to make the change of life as smooth as possible."

—Andrew Weil, M.D., Clinical Professor of Medicine
and Director, Program in Integrative Medicine,
University of Arizona

Mind Over Menopause

The Complete Mind/Body Approach
to Coping with Menopause

Leslee Kagan, M.S., N.P., Bruce Kessel, M.D.,
and Herbert Benson, M.D.

FREE PRESS
New York • London • Toronto • Sydney

*f*P

FREE PRESS
A Division of Simon & Schuster, Inc.
1230 Avenue of the Americas
New York, NY 10020

First Free Press trade paperback edition 2004

FREE PRESS and colophon are trademarks
of Simon & Schuster, Inc.

For information about special discounts for bulk purchases,
please contact Simon & Schuster Special Sales:
1-800-456-6798 or business@simonandschuster.com

Designed by Dana Sloan

Manufactured in the United States of America

1   3   5   7   9   10   8   6   4   2

Library of Congress Cataloging-in-Publication Data
Kagan, Leslee.
Mind over menopause: the complete mind/body approach to coping
with menopause / Leslee Kagan, Bruce Kessel, and Herbet Benson.
p.   cm.
Includes bibliographical references and index.
1. Menopause—Alternative treatment.   2. Mind and body—Health aspects.
3. Behavior therapy.   I. Kessel, Bruce.   II. Benson, Herbert, 1935–.   III. Title.
RG186.K34   2004
618.1'7506—dc22   2003064307

ISBN 978-0-7432-3697-3

For Leah and Eric
—LK

For Elton and Jean
—BK

For Marilyn
—HB

Contents

Contents

Acknowledgments

The ideas and advice offered in these pages reflect the integrated approach to patient care that we practice at the Mind/Body Medical Institute. We would especially like to acknowledge Eileen O'Connell, Ph.D., R.N., C.S., who dedicated so much time to recreating and adapting the menopause program in the late 1990s. We would also like to thank those colleagues who helped with key parts of this book: in particular, Ann Webster, Ph.D., and Peg Baim, M.S., N.P., for their wisdom, generosity of spirit, creative energy, enthusiasm, support, and friendship. Special thanks go to Jim Huddleston, M.S., P.T., for his expertise and work on the exercise chapter, to Marc O'Meara, R.D., for his extensive research and guidance on the nutrition chapter, and to Margie Canty, R.N., R.Y.T., and Jennifer Johnston, M.A., L.M.H.C., R.Y.T., for their contributions regarding women and yoga. We would like to acknowledge all of our colleagues at the Mind/Body Medical Institute for their pioneering work in the field of mind/body medicine, and thank them for sharing their knowledge and experiences with us, including Eva Selhub, M.D., Patti Martin Arcari, Ph.D., R.N., Janet Fronk, M.S., N.P., Ellen Slawsby, Ph.D., Carol Lynn Mandle, Ph.D., R.N., C.S., Gloria Deckro, M.D., and Aggie Casey, M.S., R.N., C.C.R.N. We would also like to acknowledge Marilyn Wilcher of the Mind/Body Medical Institute, whose support and wise guidance contributed to the smooth evolution of this work. In addition, we extend much gratitude to Marcie K.

Richardson, M.D., an expert in the field of women's health and menopause, for her invaluable insight in reviewing the manuscript.

We are deeply indebted to Kristin DeJohn for her unwavering dedication, creative guidance, intelligence, and sensitivity in helping to write this book, and thus make it a reality. We offer warm thanks to Alice D. Domar, Ph.D., for having the vision to suggest a series of books on mind/body medicine and for her insightful comments about this manuscript. We would also like to thank our colleagues at Harvard Medical School. Anthony Komaroff, M.D., editor in chief at Harvard Health Publications, provided invaluable editorial guidance while we wrote. Edward Coburn, publishing director, with the assistance of Nancy Ferrari, managing editor, and assistant editors Joan McGrath and Christine Junge, provided encouragement, resources, and an editorial approach, which kept us focused on the reader's needs.

To our families:

I, Leslee Kagan, would like to express my love and gratitude to my children, Leah and Eric, the two joys of my life. Their patience and understanding enabled me to take the time I needed to write this book. I also want to express my thanks to my sister, Marcy Kagan, for her unconditional love and compassion, to my mother, Matile Kagan, who believed I could do this, and to Jeff Riklin for lending a helping hand.

I, Herbert Benson, am forever grateful to my wife, Marilyn.

I, Bruce Kessel, express my love for my parents, Elton and Jean Kessel.

Finally, we would like to thank our patients for their willingness to share their stories. Many of the women we have worked with have been an inspiration. Overcoming tough times, they have gone on to embrace the best of life and, in the process, transform their journey. We hope you, too, will follow in their footsteps—finding health, happiness, and a zest for life.

LESLEE KAGAN, M.S., N.P.

BRUCE KESSEL, M.D.

HERBERT BENSON, M.D.

Mind Over Menopause

Introduction

Throughout life we are faced with many pathways. It is the paths we choose that affect how we live and the way we feel. Some women see midlife as a crossroads—a time of change and potential. This can be a truly exhilarating time for women who embrace possibilities and maintain their health. It can be a time of profound growth and creative endeavor—a time to strengthen social bonds and tap into inner wisdom.

The menopause transition is a unique experience for each woman. Many women cruise through it with few problems. But the transition can throw up some real physiological "speed bumps." The erratic nature of fluctuating hormones during this time can make life difficult and for some women extremely trying. These are the women who walk through our doors. They often complain of difficulty sleeping, troubling hot flashes, mood swings, worsening PMS, concerns about memory, and difficulty managing menopausal symptoms within the context of their busy lives. They may experience feelings of isolation. Concerns about sexuality and other changes may be affecting their interpersonal relationships. Often, sharing their stories and talking about the transition with other women makes a big difference. As they learn more, they soon find that they have more control over how they feel than they had originally thought possible.

If you notice that hormonal fluctuations are affecting the way you feel or slowing you down, you are *not* alone! And you are not alone if you are apprehensive about which path to take when it comes to medical care. Debates over hormone use have left many women unsure of what to do and whom to trust.

In *Mind Over Menopause,* we hope to help you sort through your many health care options. Most importantly, we hope to convince you that *you* are your best guide. You hold the power when it comes to knowing your body, understanding your symptoms, and determining your needs. And you'd be surprised at how much power you have in managing the midlife transition.

What we have found, based on thirty-five years of research and patient care, is that we all possess an innate ability to heal and overcome adversity in both a physical and an emotional sense. The years around menopause are a great time to reassess your health care; tend to your physical, emotional, and spiritual needs; and look toward the future. Our goal is to provide helpful advice about how you can make changes, starting today, which will help you manage the symptoms of menopause and improve your long-term health.

The strategies we describe, "tools" as we like to call them, are the same ones that we offer to patients in our Mind Over Menopause Program at the Mind/Body Medical Institute. The basic program lasts for ten weeks, during which time participants attend weekly two-and-a-half-hour sessions. The first program was developed in 1991 by Alice Domar, Ph.D., and was refined and enhanced by Eileen O'Connell, Ph.D., R.N., C.S., in 1997. Under the guidance of Leslee Kagan, M.S., N.P., it has continued to grow—helping many women make significant changes in their lives and ease or eliminate their symptoms.

One of our groups was evaluated in a pilot study in 1999, and the results were presented to the North American Menopause Society—a scientific, nonprofit organization devoted to promoting women's health during midlife and beyond. When the participants were tested after the program concluded, they were found to have experienced substantial improvements in their quality of life. Their hot flashes were reduced in intensity and number, they experienced marked reductions in psychological distress, including depression, and they felt more prepared to manage their "stressors." They were also more comfortable talking about issues and found great support in empathizing with other women. As a result, they felt less isolated and more connected.

In addition to these improvements, these women had been successful in adopting a variety of health-promoting behaviors. Months after their participation, they were still exercising more, eating better, and experiencing enhanced personal relationships and spiritual growth. All told, the pilot study demonstrated that this is a healthy, self-care approach to menopause, one that could not be accomplished by a prescription alone!

We believe you too can benefit from the many tools we teach.

In this book, you will find a step-by-step guide to managing menopause that combines the latest information about stress management, nutrition, exercise, and other health care decisions, including an approach to medications. This book builds on advice offered in earlier books by Dr. Herbert Benson, particularly *The Relaxation Response* and *The Wellness Book*. It also builds on the work done by Alice D. Domar, Ph.D., who applied these teachings to women's health issues and passed her knowledge on to readers in her books *Self-Nurture* and *Healing Mind, Healthy Woman*. Mind Over Menopause is just one of several clinical programs that are offered at the Mind/Body Medical Institute. We also have programs to help people deal with heart disease, infertility, insomnia, cancer, HIV, chronic pain, and general stress-related symptoms. Founded in 1988 at Beth Israel Deaconess Medical Center, the Mind/Body Medical Institute is a nonprofit organization dedicated to advancing scientific research, public education, and professional training in the field of mind/body medicine. This field helps people tap their own natural capacity to heal in a way that complements other traditional medical approaches. At the Mind/Body Medical Institute, we employ an interdisciplinary team of exercise physiologists, advanced practice nurses, dietitians, psychologists, and physicians who together have developed the strategies you will find in this book. Thousands of people have already completed our mind/body programs, and made significant changes in their lives. We hope you can use the tools and knowledge in this book as you embark on your journey.

A variety of health professionals may play important roles in the care of menopausal women. These providers range from physicians to nurse practitioners, from psychologists to nutritionists. For this reason, we've used the term *clinician* throughout the book to refer to those individuals providing clinical care to menopausal women.

Note: Patients' names have been changed throughout to preserve confidentiality.

CHAPTER 1

Redefining "The Change"

Imagine hovering at the edge of a lake. You know the water is going to be cold, but you ease in (or maybe you plunge in headfirst!). At first it's unbearable, but as you work your muscles, the discomfort goes away and you enjoy the swim. For many women, menopause is like this. The transition can be difficult and there may be apprehension, but when all is said and done, it's not as bad as expected. They may even walk away feeling invigorated and full of life.

Millions of women worldwide report the years after menopause as a time of increased confidence and feelings of empowerment. As Margaret Mead, one of the world's foremost anthropologists, observed, "There is no more creative force in the world than the menopausal woman with zest."

And, that creative force is growing exponentially. The aging of the "baby boomers" means that an unprecedented number of women are reaching menopause now. In the United States, there are approximately 42 million women over the age of fifty. From 1990 to 2030, some 1.2 billion women worldwide will go through the years of "the change." As millions of women look for meaning and seek answers, menopause is truly being redefined. It is long overdue.

Menopause and Beyond

A century ago, most women did not live much beyond the age of menopause. But today, a woman who is healthy at menopause can expect to live another thirty or forty years. That's more than a third of your life! And unlike past generations, women now speak openly about menopause. The increase in communication has come at an important time. Today women are faced with more choices about their health care than ever before. Making good choices regarding lifestyle and health care can help you fill your postmenopausal years with happiness and health.

Menopausal symptoms, heart disease, and osteoporosis are all major concerns for women at midlife because all are linked to declining levels of the hormone estrogen. One of the biggest decisions in the past—and probably the most confusing—has been whether or not to take hormones. Yet research is proving estrogen is only part of a much larger and complex equation, still not entirely understood.

What is becoming increasingly evident is that the way we feel, how we handle symptoms, and our risk for disease are dramatically linked to our lifestyles. The advice we offer in this book is the same that we provide to participants in our mind/body program for menopause called Mind Over Menopause. The framework for all of our programs is based on the philosophy that your attitudes, health care choices, and lifestyle behaviors can significantly affect your overall well-being. Some women enter our programs simply seeking information to help them make decisions. Some express sadness at the loss of their youth and are looking for ways to change their perceptions of getting older. Others want the tools to manage menopause symptoms. And still others seek support from women facing similar life-stage issues.

The techniques and advice we offer in this book are designed to give you the power to manage menopause symptoms while reducing your long-term risk for disease. They have been backed by scientific research, and women in our programs have found them to make a profound difference in the quality of their lives. Our patients report a decrease in intensity of hot flashes, improved sleep, a significant decrease in tension and anxiety, and a decrease in depression. In addition, they are successful at making long-lasting changes in their health habits. However, none of the information in this book is designed to supplant advice from your clinician. Rather, we hope it will help you ask the right questions, make informed decisions, and move through this transition smoothly as you build a foundation for lasting health.

A Natural Transition

Contrary to popular belief, menopause is not a medical problem that requires treatment. It is a natural biological event that marks the permanent end to your menstrual periods and, thus, of your childbearing years. It is not a disease and, for the majority of women, does not require medical intervention.

When you've gone a full year without a menstrual period, you've officially reached menopause. Some women will hit this stage in their forties, some in their late fifties. The average age of natural menopause in the Western world is fifty-one. But menopause can occur naturally at an earlier age or can be induced as a result of surgery, radiation, or chemotherapy.

The transitional time leading up to natural menopause is called perimenopause. During this time, which can span several years, the production of hormones that have regulated your cycles for years becomes erratic. Jumps and starts can cause you to experience subtle and not so subtle changes related to these fluctuating hormones. It's this changing and often unpredictable hormonal milieu that sets the stage for symptoms like hot flashes, night sweats, headaches, and mood swings.

For many women, symptoms are mild; for others, they interfere substantially with daily life. Each woman's experience of this transition is unique. And how you feel is not simply a matter of hormone levels. Biology plays a role, but so do the interactions among your mind, body, and environment.

The Mind/Body Link

The term "mind/body" refers to the many complicated interactions that take place between your thoughts, your body, and the outside world. It is based on the idea that our thoughts, attitudes, and lifestyle choices play a major role in our overall health.

Mind/body medicine, also known as behavioral medicine, got its start in the late 1960s when Dr. Herbert Benson, joined by other researchers, provided the first convincing scientific evidence that it was possible to alter the physiology of the body simply by quieting the mind. At the time, Dr. Benson was working with colleagues at Harvard Medical School to determine the cause of high blood pressure. During the study several practitioners of transcendental meditation arrived at the center claiming that they could lower their own blood pressure by meditating. Such ideas were met with skepticism in the medical community. Few believed there was even a link between stress and high blood pressure.

Dr. Benson eventually agreed to take a series of physiological measurements to determine the effects of meditation on the body. Meanwhile, a separate team of doctors in California was simultaneously conducting similar experiments. Both teams reached similar conclusions: meditation slows heart rate and breathing, reduces metabolism, lowers blood pressure, and even changes the type of brain waves generated. The findings paved the way for a great deal of insight into how the mind affects the body. It prompted Dr. Benson to describe a phenomenon he called the relaxation response (RR), a physical, natural state that is the opposite of a state of stress. (See Chapter 3 for information on how to elicit the relaxation response.)

The Many Faces of Stress

You may have heard of the fight-or-flight response. This stress response enables us to escape a threatening or dangerous situation by fighting or running. Heart rate and blood pressure increase dramatically, and adrenaline and other hormones surge through the body.

In daily life, various stresses challenge us. It is estimated that many of us trigger some type of stress response up to fifty times a day. Simply thinking about a stressful or threatening event can trigger the same chemical cascade. Scientists have demonstrated that up to a certain point, stress is useful and helps us take the action to perform necessary tasks. Harvard researchers Robert Yerkes and John Dodson have observed that as stress and anxiety increase, so do performance and efficiency—up to a point. When stress becomes chronic or excessive, the body becomes unable to adapt and cope, and stress becomes *dis*tress. Not surprisingly, many of us have passed the point of "efficient" stress. We rarely face the truly life-threatening situations for which the fight-or-flight response was intended. The problem is that repeated stress without rest can have significant physical, psychological, and behavioral consequences. For women going through menopause, it is linked to symptoms like hot flashes, insomnia, headaches, and mood swings. It also increases the risk for long-term diseases like heart disease.

The Benefits of the Relaxation Response (RR)

Fortunately, the relaxation response is the physiological antithesis of the fight-or-flight response and counters stress. This innate response decreases metabolism, heart rate, blood pressure, breathing rate, and muscle tension. Research shows that, when practiced regularly, the RR not only counteracts the harmful effects of stress on a daily basis, but it also has a "carryover" effect. It can actually make you more resilient to stress over the long term.

The findings about meditation and the relaxation response were just the first in a series of exciting insights into how the mind affects the body and vice versa. And while the field of mind/body medicine has evolved significantly in the last forty years, its basic premise remains straightforward: maintaining good health requires that you attend to your mind as well as your body. Negative thoughts and moods can affect you physically, just as hot flashes, lack of sleep, and stiff joints and muscles can affect you emotionally. Quiet the mind and you can calm the body; quiet the body and you can calm the mind.

Balancing Your Health

Since the mid-twentieth century, when antibiotics were discovered, Western medicine has come to rely heavily on interventions like medicine and surgery. In this approach to health, the patient comes to the doctor and the doctor does something to make her better. Harvard health psychologist Dr. Ann Webster characterizes this model of medicine in the following way:

- Patient is a passive recipient of the doctor's care.
- Doctors are believed to know more than the patient.
- Patient cooperates, follows instructions, and doesn't ask many questions.

This is the "find it and fix it" model most of us grew up with. We may remember our mothers simply doing as their doctors told them without giving much input or expecting many answers. This old model of health care, while tempting to follow, is inadequate in today's complex world. As a paradigm shift takes hold of the medical world, women by the millions are now realizing the time for a proactive approach to health care is long overdue.

In the mind/body model of health care, we view health as a partnership that may require important medical and surgical interventions, but we also value *self-care* as an equally important component in maintaining overall health. In this more comprehensive approach, you become an integral player in the outcome of your health care. In Dr. Webster's words:

- Healing is shared; all caregivers do their part.
- Patients are partners in the treatment decisions and understand what is necessary for health and well-being.
- Self-care is important: Patients care about themselves enough to make alterations in lifestyle and health habits.
- Patients access their own inner resources for healing as a supplement to other forms of treatment.

Dr. Benson has described this more comprehensive approach of treatment by using the metaphor of a three-legged stool to represent the proper balance needed in order to achieve optimal health. One leg of the stool consists of the use of medications to prevent and treat diseases. Surgical interventions and procedures represent the second leg. The third leg of the stool, self-care, signifies the strategies you use to enhance your own natural capacity to heal.

The third leg includes the relaxation response, exercise, nutrition, cognitive approaches (learning to use your thoughts to serve you better), and any belief that promotes health, including spirituality. The concept of self-care involves being good to your body, mind, and soul. In short, it encompasses anything you can do to affect your general health in a positive way.

The Three-Legged Stool

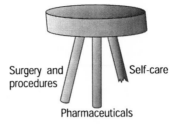

Surgery and procedures

Self-care

Pharmaceuticals

While all three legs of the stool have been verified through scientific research, all too often, patients and clinicians ignore the third leg of self-care. Disregarding self-care—what you can do to promote your health—can result in a health care approach that is as wobbly and off-balance as, well, a two-legged stool.

The bottom line is that you can have the best clinicians and facilities in the world, yet they will not guarantee good health. A stunning example of this is the health scenario in the United States. A comparison of health care costs in twenty-three industrialized countries found that the United States spent the most money, yet ranked second to last when it came to healthy life expectancy. (Japan ranked first in life expectancy, followed by Switzerland.)

In 1979, the U.S. surgeon general issued a report that stated that as many as half the premature deaths in this country could be attributable to unhealthy behaviors or lifestyles (lack of self-care). It further suggested that, of the ten leading causes of premature death, at least seven could be substantially reduced if Americans altered their bad habits. These habits included poor diet, smoking, lack of exercise, alcohol abuse, and unhealthy responses to tension and stress.

Today, more than twenty years later, more people are out of shape and unhealthy than ever before. It is estimated that 61 percent of adults in the United States are overweight or obese. Diabetes rates are soaring. Health care costs are rising. Yet many people are in denial or simply unaware that their lifestyles affect the way they feel and how long they will live. By embracing self-care, you can maximize your health and improve the quality of your life—and manage menopause symptoms while you're at it. The best part is that many women truly enjoy the process.

Self-Care and Menopause

During the years around menopause, most women know instinctively that their bodies are changing. Learning to pay attention to what is happening and to describe what you're experiencing to your health care provider is an important part of self-care. It is key to getting the help you need, and by working in partnership with your clinician, you become an active participant. This puts you in the position to fully understand your options and make choices that feel right for you. After all, knowledge is power!

In our programs, we teach women that by building awareness they can feel more in control and more effectively manage their menopause symptoms, and ultimately their overall health. What you eat, how much you exercise, and the nature of your interactions with other people all affect your health. It is in building awareness that women begin to recognize what they need, and make changes necessary to improve their health and well-being. If you've noticed that stress affects symptoms like hot flashes and insomnia, or that when you exercise you feel happier, then you've already begun to understand the basis for the mind/body connection.

The goal of many of the exercises in this book is to help you develop the awareness that can lead to change. Doing the three-column stress awareness exercise (see sidebar, page 14), Ruth began to recognize early stress warnings, which has helped her avoid unnecessary aggravation. In her words: "I became very clear and very focused on

An Awareness-Building Exercise

Grab a pencil and paper and try this exercise.

1. Make three columns on your paper and title them: "Stressor," "How stress makes me feel," and "How I react when I am stressed."
2. In the first column list the kinds of things that create stress in your life (for example, juggling work and family, commuting).
3. In the second column describe your physical and emotional responses to these stressors (for example, neck stiffens, anxiety increases).
4. In the third column list what you do in reaction to the stressors (for example, eat, smoke, yell).

Column/List #1: Some common stressors for women in our programs include balancing work and home life, kids, commuting, finances, work/boss, and family relationships. (Yours may vary.)

Column #2: Women report that these stressors make them anxious, irritable, depressed, and cause them to have headaches, difficulty sleeping, stiff necks and shoulders, painful jaws, heart palpitations, difficulty concentrating, and more frequent hot flashes.

Column #3: Their common ways to cope include losing their temper, overeating, shopping, smoking, drinking, talking to a friend, taking a walk, and counting to ten.

what my warning signals were. For me it was a racing heart. Then I might become aware of a tightening in the back of my throat or in my stomach. And I began to see the pattern. Instead of letting it escalate to the point that I would feel sick, I now take time out to do breathing exercises. It's the difference between night and day. If you can cut stress off at the pass before it really begins to escalate, then you can much more successfully control it. You never hit that adrenaline high that can make you feel really ill and totally stressed out." By incorporating a range of mind/body skills, Ruth was able to more effectively

STRESSORS

In column one, you've identified your stressors. We have no control over many of the stressors in our lives, but we do have control over our *responses* to them and our *perceptions* of their meanings. When you can change your perceptions, you can change the way you respond. (See Chapter 10 for information on how to do this.)

STRESS WARNING SIGNS

By describing how these stressors make you feel in column two, you've identified your personal stress warning signs. They are akin to the little red light on the dashboard of your car that warns that the engine is overheating and if you don't do something to intervene, it will blow. These symptoms are the physical and psychological consequences of stress. Although taken by themselves they may not appear serious, if these warning signs are ignored and allowed to continue, they can lead to serious illnesses such as heart disease and high blood pressure. Luckily, they can be effectively dealt with using the stress-reducing techniques we teach.

COPING STRATEGIES

Column three represents your current strategies for coping with your stress. Some of these may be healthy coping behaviors (counting to ten, talking to a friend), and some of these may be unhealthy (smoking, drinking, using drugs, etc). Although the latter may feel good in the moment, in the long run they will adversely affect your health. Our goal is to add to your list of healthy coping skills.

manage stress, improve communication with her family, and reduce hot flashes and other menopause-related symptoms.

Throughout this book, we will offer you the skills and knowledge that will help you not only listen to your body, but also change the way you feel. Many women meet menopause head on with a strength and vitality that is unparalleled. With the right tools, you can too.

Your Body on Stress

Have you ever noticed that when you're stressed or tense, your posture and muscles change? To get a better idea of how stress affects your body, try this exercise:

1. Place your arm out in front of you.
2. Make a fist, clenching tightly and count to five.
3. Focus on your breath: What happens to your breathing?

You may have noticed that you temporarily held your breath. You might not realize it, but you likely do this throughout the day. Shallow, ineffective breathing is common. When we carry around stress and tension, they affect us in many ways. (For tips on how to improve breathing and reduce stress, see Chapter 3.)

CHAPTER 2

Understanding Hormonal Changes

If you've ever watched the ocean over a period of time, you understand the concept of cycles. Nature is cyclical and we are cyclical beings. Even a good night's sleep depends on our ability to stay "in sync" with daylight cycles and our environment. With this in mind, think about how our bodies are regulated. A complex network of hormones and other chemicals are all hardwired to keep us alive and well. Some keep us safe, others keep us happy, and yet others are in charge of creation.

What makes this so complex? While each chemical has a certain job, its movement and presence directly affect other body systems. Like the tides, the ebb and flow of female hormones typically fall into regular cycles during our childbearing years. Female hormones direct the menstrual cycle, make it possible to become pregnant, and make women look different from men. Beautifully designed to create life, the female body is also an exquisitely sensitive system.

Normal cycles rely on the intricate interplay of hormones, which affects not only our menstrual cycles, but also distant parts of the body. Regardless of age, each woman responds differently to hormonal changes. That means each woman's experience of the menopausal transition is unique. For some, it creates barely a ripple. For others it summons waves. And, for a part of the female population, it feels more like an approaching storm! As you consider and experience the physical changes associated with menopause, keep in mind that this is a natural and normal phase of life. To better understand these changes, it is helpful to understand your body, how hormones affect you, and why.

The word "hormone," derived from the Greek word for "messenger," is a fitting name. Hormones travel through our bodies influencing how we move, how we think, and how we behave. Sent from hormone-producing glands in the body, as well as the brain, they are influenced by our biology and our environment.

Both sexes share many hormones, but they arise in acutely different levels to carry out different functions. The dominant female hormones, produced by the ovaries, are estrogen, progesterone, and testosterone. They travel throughout the body, from the brain to the vagina. Along the route, each hormone interacts with specific receptors. Like a key, if a hormone has the correct "fit," it interacts with that receptor and creates an action. For example, estrogen on a certain pathway acts to build up the lining of the uterus. In other areas of the body, it may help protect bone. Because estrogen receptors are abundant throughout the body, changing levels of estrogen can affect many organ systems, including those involved in reproduction as well as the heart, bones, and brain.

Menstrual Cycles:
The Hormonal Dance

Women are born with all of their eggs, one to two million of them, in their ovaries. Each egg is contained in a tiny sac called a follicle. Through childhood, the follicles remain dormant. But as we near puberty, the system gears up for a dramatic change. We don't know exactly what triggers puberty, but we do know that it's the beginning of a complex system of hormonal shifts that will mark our reproductive years. At puberty, the ovaries begin to produce estrogen. This pri-

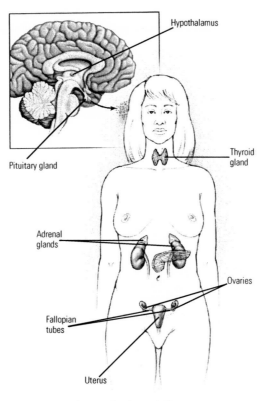

Hormone Production in Women

mary female hormone is a key messenger in the hormonal cascade that ripens the egg and releases it from the follicle (ovulation).

Once an egg is released, the ovaries add progesterone to the estrogen mix. This prepares the body for pregnancy. Estrogen causes the lining of the uterus to grow. Progesterone causes changes in the lining that will allow an embryo to implant and, thereby, allow a pregnancy to begin. In short, both perform critical roles. If a pregnancy does not occur, estrogen and progesterone levels fall. The uterus sheds its lining in preparation for starting the cycle over again. This is the menstrual period.

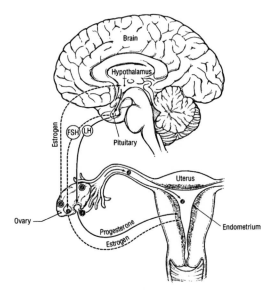

The Hormonal Dance

The hypothalamus area of the brain directs the hormonal system. It is influenced by many external factors, including emotions, stress, and diet, as well as hormones from other parts of the reproductive system. The hypothalamus secretes gonadotropin-releasing hormone (GnRH), which signals the nearby pituitary gland to produce follicle-stimulating hormone (FSH) and luteinizing hormone (LH). These enter the bloodstream and, when they reach the ovaries, stimulate the growth of a follicle containing an egg cell, and trigger ovulation. After ovulation, the ovaries produce higher levels of progesterone and estradiol, which promote endometrial growth in the uterus. If no pregnancy ensues, hormone levels fall and you get your menstrual period, resetting the hypothalamus/pituitary cycle.

To lead this complex orchestration, you need a conductor. That would be the hypothalamus, a small area in the base of the brain. The hypothalamus directs cycles by sending hormones that tell the nearby pituitary gland to release FSH (follicle-stimulating hormone) and LH (luteinizing hormone). Both are important in ensuring regular ovulatory cycles. They stimulate the ovary, which causes a follicle to "mature," and they trigger ovulation. During our reproductive years, many factors like stress, hunger, and danger can affect our systems by triggering surges of chemicals that can disrupt the natural cycle.

Perimenopause: A Midlife Transition

As nature would have it, the body wasn't meant to have babies indefinitely. When a woman reaches perimenopause, she has substantially fewer egg-containing follicles remaining in her ovaries. The follicles that do remain respond poorly to the signals of FSH and LH. Pregnancy is still possible, but ovulation and menstrual periods usually become irregular.

Ironically, while menopause is associated with *lower* levels of female hormones, perimenopause can actually be a time of *increased* levels. As the follicles become less responsive to FSH, the pituitary gland responds by cranking out larger amounts of this hormone to "wake up" the ovary and achieve ovulation. During some cycles, an ovary will respond by triggering the production of higher levels of estrogen, and ovulation will occur. In other cycles the ovary does not respond. It is this often erratic fluctuation of hormones that is a defining characteristic of this part of the transition.

Erratic ovulation disrupts the normally very cyclical ebb and flow of estrogen and progesterone. Although not completely understood, menopause symptoms appear to correlate with fluctuating hormone levels. It is believed that when estrogen levels are high, a woman may have symptoms such as breast tenderness. When estro-

Common Perimenopausal Complaints

- Changes in menstrual cycle: shortening or lengthening of menstrual cycles; skipped or irregular periods; periods that are more painful, lighter, or heavier than usual
- PMS getting worse or happening for the first time
- Hot flashes
- Night sweats
- Insomnia
- Irritability, mood swings, depressive symptoms
- Fatigue
- Headaches
- Vaginal dryness/decreased lubrication
- Concerns about memory and ability to concentrate
- Sexual response changes
- Muscle/joint aches and pains

gen levels fall, she may notice hot flashes and vaginal dryness or irritation. As estrogen rapidly cycles from high to low levels, it may result in mood swings or PMS (premenstrual syndrome, a constellation of physical and psychological symptoms that appear prior to menses and resolve after). For many women, the appearance or worsening of PMS may be one of the first signs of perimenopause.

Riding the Waves

Many women glide through the menopause transition with relatively few problems. But, for others, changing hormonal tides can bring a maelstrom of symptoms. Because these symptoms are often unpredictable, many women also feel a loss of control, which adds to the difficulty. Imagine being a captain of a boat and not knowing when to expect low tide.

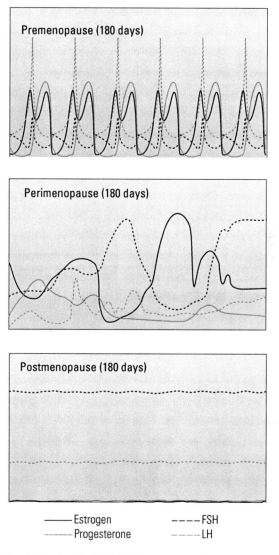

Hormones During Regular Menstrual Cycles, the Perimenopause, and Menopause

Measurements of estrogen, progesterone, FSH (follicle stimulating hormone), and LH (luteinizing hormone) show the erratic nature of their levels during perimenopause compared with both premenopause and post-menopause.

For Lee, the first signs of perimenopause came in her forties. "I began having my period every three weeks. It was completely draining and it was hard to figure out when to expect problems," she recalls. "I felt as if I didn't have control of my body."

Perimenopause is often compared to a roller coaster. Many women cannot tell when the twists, turns, and free falls will happen. Some compare the perimenopausal transition to the highs and lows of puberty. From a scientific standpoint, the hormonal fluctuations during puberty and those seen during perimenopause are actually quite similar. Fortunately, for those women who do feel at the mercy of their hormones, there is good news. The "ride" does not go on forever.

After perimenopause, hormones level off. The transition from perimenopause to postmenopause is one that is defined in retrospect. A woman at midlife is considered to have reached menopause after one full year without any menstrual periods.

Menopause: "The Change"

As a woman eases out of the transition into menopause, the hormonal highs and lows begin to disappear and estrogen levels stabilize, although at a lower level. This often relieves many symptoms of perimenopause, such as mood changes, irregular periods, and headaches. Hot flashes may continue, however, and symptoms related to low estrogen levels, such as vaginal dryness, may worsen.

Overall, the leveling off of hormones can actually make menopause a bit of a relief. "When I reached my early fifties, the problems really went away," says Lee. "I had some hot flashes, but I don't recall them being too bothersome." For many women, freedom from menstrual cycles can be a good thing. It can make life a bit easier, and with birth control no longer a consideration many women enjoy a newfound sexual freedom. Psychologically, this can be a time of profound growth, challenges, and opportunities.

In 1998, the North American Menopause Society polled 752 women between ages fifty and sixty-five. They were asked, "In which period of your life did you feel the most content or were you the happiest?" Fifty-one percent reported being most content after age fifty. Only 16 percent chose their forties, 17 percent their thirties, and 10 percent their twenties as the period in which they were the most content and happy.

How Do You Know It's Menopause?

One of the first questions a woman asks when noticing changes linked to menopause is: "What is happening to my body?" Dana, thinking back to when she was thirty-nine, now realizes she was probably experiencing the beginning of perimenopause. She had noticed mild, infrequent hot flashes, but wrote them off to illness or fatigue. "I didn't realize at the time that that's what it was," she recalls. "It had crossed my mind, but I thought, 'oh, I'm too young.' " As the years passed, night sweats would come in spells, then disappear for months.

Cheryl also recalls that her symptoms started subtly and lasted for many years. She became increasingly intolerant of heat of any kind. When she had her first hot flash, she simply did not know what it was. She also began having mood swings and cramps. "People used to just call it PMS. I think a lot of women are now realizing it's the beginning of perimenopause."

So how can you tell whether irregular periods, hot flashes, PMS, or insomnia are signs of perimenopause or something else?

The "menopause test": Right now, there is no reliable test for perimenopause. Some clinicians may recommend a blood test to look for high levels of FSH (follicle stimulating hormone). But this test isn't reliable because FSH levels, like estrogen levels, often rise and fall unpredictably during the menopause transition. Because FSH levels can vary from month to month, a single test may not be enough. Also, when the blood sample is tested at a random time during the menstrual cycle, a "normal" result can be misleading and be misinterpreted to mean that a woman's symptoms are *not* linked to menopause. This can leave many women feeling as though "it's all in their heads." If an FSH level is recommended, it should be drawn on the third day of the menstrual cycle. Elevated FSH levels on this day have been shown to correlate with diminished fertility, which can be an indication of perimenopause.

Tracking symptoms: There may not be a clear-cut test for perimenopause, but you can track important changes that you notice. Is your menstrual cycle noticeably different from a few years ago? Is your cycle shorter or your flow heavier? The answers to these questions will help you and your clinician determine whether you might be entering perimenopause.

Early on, your menstrual cycle may shorten, with periods beginning sooner than you expect. Maybe your periods used to come every twenty-eight days. Now, they come every twenty-three days. Any pattern is possible. Bleeding also may become lighter or heavier. Keep a calendar to record changes. The more accurately you can describe symptoms and irregularities, the easier it will be to pinpoint changes related to perimenopause.

Ruling out other medical conditions

Changes in patterns of uterine bleeding can present a confusing picture. If you are fifty-two years old, have stopped having periods and are experiencing hot flashes and night sweats, these changes are probably due to menopause. But what if you are thirty-five years old, have stopped having periods, and don't have hot flashes? This requires further evaluation including testing for early menopause, thyroid prob-

					Final menstrual period		
Stages of reproductive aging					**0**		
Stage	-5	-4	-3	-2	-1	+1	+2
	Reproductive years			Perimenopause		Postmenopause	
	Early	Peak	Late	Early	Late	Early	Late
Menstrual cycle	Variable to regular	Regular		Variable	Skipped periods	None	
Follicle stimulating hormone (FSH)	Normal FSH			Elevated FSH			

Reproductive aging

Sometimes it seems women live three lives in one: childhood, the reproductive years, and postmenopause. Recently, experts in women's health and aging put forth the concept that these are part of an ongoing physiological process that they call "reproductive aging."

Simply put, reproductive aging is what happens to the ovaries and other reproductive organs as women age. In July 2001, a group of twenty-seven experts in aging and women's health met in Park City, Utah, for the Stages of Reproductive Aging Workshop (STRAW). Their goal was to describe this process in greater detail. To do this, they divided the process into seven stages, beginning with the early years of the menstrual cycle and continuing for the remainder of a woman's life. All seven stages describe in simple terms what happens to menstrual cycles and levels of follicle stimulating hormone as a woman ages.

The staging system doesn't specifically outline when and to what levels estrogen and other reproductive hormones decline because these changes are extremely variable among individual women. Experts emphasize that not all healthy women will follow these stages sequentially—some women may skip some of the stages—and the age range during which they occur can vary widely.

What is the point of this staging system? Eventually, experts hope it wil help women and their physicians determine where in the reproductive aging process a woman is so that appropriate care can be given. This approach is new, and many clinicians aren't familiar with it yet. Besides helping to improve medical care for midlife women, experts hope the staging system will help direct biomedical researchers to fill in many of the current knowledge gaps about menopause.

lems, pregnancy, or an increase in the hormone prolactin (which can suppress ovulation). Some women stop having menstrual periods during their reproductive years because of a condition called *functional hypothalamic amenorrhea*. A combination of stress, weight loss, and excessive exercise is usually behind this problem.

Abnormal bleeding may also be a sign of abnormalities within the uterus (polyps, fibroids, precancerous changes, or uterine cancer). So it's important to keep track of changes in bleeding patterns and discuss them with your clinician. If these uterine conditions have been ruled out, irregular menstrual cycles may be related to perimenopause and can be treated with a variety of medications including birth control pills and progesterone.

Premature and induced menopause

Premature (or early) *menopause* is defined as menopause that occurs before age forty (this is an arbitrary cutoff point). Management of symptoms may be similar, but the risks and benefits of hormone therapy are likely to stack up differently. Women who experience early menopause have an increased lifetime risk for developing osteoporosis, possibly heart disease and urogenital problems. This is because they live more of their lives without the protective effects of estrogen. The benefits of hormone replacement therapy in this situation may outweigh the risks.

Induced menopause means that the ovaries have been removed surgically or damaged (usually due to chemotherapy or radiation therapy). This may or may not have been done as part of a hysterectomy (removal of the uterus only).

A hysterectomy usually does not cause immediate menopause, although periods cease after surgery. The ovaries remain in the body and eventually undergo the hormonal shifts of menopause. However, some women who have this procedure may experience menopause within a few years of the operation, regardless of their age and despite the fact that the ovaries haven't been removed. When a woman has her uterus *and* both ovaries removed, she will experience "menopause" immediately. Symptoms may be more dramatic than those of women whose menopause occurs "naturally."

Induced menopause is generally much tougher for women than natural menopause. Levels of all ovarian hormones (estrogen, progesterone, testosterone, and adrostendione) drop rapidly. Symptoms (hot flashes and mood) may be more severe, and sex drive (libido), which is influenced by testosterone, may be affected. Extreme hot flashes can begin immediately.

Quality of life issues, the age of induced menopause, and the reason it occurred are all considerations in deciding treatment options. Hormones are usually indicated for short-term symptom relief. The scale may be tipped in favor of long-term use if a woman is young.

Unique menopausal concerns of women with breast cancer

Women with a history of breast cancer deal with at least four specific issues related to menopause:

- The possibility of induced menopause either as a result of removal of the ovaries or ovarian damage due to chemotherapy
- A general reluctance by clinicians and patients to use estrogen following a diagnosis of breast cancer, because some breast cancers are estrogen sensitive (meaning that the presence of estrogen in the body may promote the cancer)
- The possible use of tamoxifen (used to treat breast cancer) that may worsen some menopausal symptoms (particularly hot flashes)
- The effects of chemotherapy and radiation on quality of life

Breast cancer patients are often unprepared for the issues surrounding induced menopause, including the potential loss of their fertility and the possible abrupt onset of menopausal symptoms.

Ann was only forty-one when she was diagnosed with breast cancer. Her entire life turned upside down: "I had just lost a breast. I was thrown into this hormone maelstrom. Then all of a sudden I had vaginal issues and a lack of sex drive. I was totally unprepared." On top of this, Ann was prescribed tamoxifen after her surgery. "I didn't realize that the tamoxifen would cause hot flashes," she recalls. "I'd get these feelings of anxiety before the hot flash. So when it first happened, I thought I was going out of my mind." Many women share her experience. Information and support can greatly enhance a woman's ability to adjust and cope. A teamwork approach to treatment is best, incorporating perspectives from both oncologists and gynecologists.

Menopause and a medical partnership

Menopause is a natural transition and does not necessarily require medical intervention. But some women find that their symptoms af-

Finding a Menopause "Specialist"

Unlike other medical specialties, there is no board certification in "menopause." But practitioners across a number of medical disciplines have taken a special interest in menopause.

- *Family practice doctors and internists:* These physicians all have training in women's health.
- *Nurse practitioners (NPs)/nurse midwives (CNMs):* Nurse practitioners and midwives have often developed special interest areas in women's health, including menopause.
- *Obstetricians/gynecologists (Ob/Gyns):* These physicians have extensive training in a broad range of women's health issues including menopause.
- *Reproductive endocrinologists:* These doctors are ob/gyns with an additional three years of training in reproductive endocrinology and infertility. They all have expertise with regard to menopause, and a substantial number concentrate exclusively on research and/or clinical care of midlife women.
- *Menopause centers/women's centers:* A menopause center that is part of a teaching hospital/medical school is likely to be an excellent resource.

The North American Menopause Society (NAMS) is a nonprofit organization dedicated to the science of menopause and improving quality of life for women at midlife and beyond. It provides referral lists of its members in the United States and Canada (go to www.menopause.org). The list includes clinicians who are members of the society, as well as those who have passed a NAMS competency exam in menopause.

fect their quality of life. If that's true for you and you're considering treatment, think of your relationship with your clinician as a working partnership. Learn about menopause, know your family history, and go into your appointments with a sense of how you want to approach things. If you do not wish to take medications, be prepared to discuss lifestyle options. It's important that the clinician you choose addresses your concerns and respects your viewpoint. Ask yourself the following questions:

- Am I being listened to?
- Are my concerns being taken seriously or dismissed? If so, does this happen often?
- Am I comfortable discussing personal health issues, including sexuality?
- Are my values and concerns regarding treatment respected?
- Do I feel confident in the clinician's knowledge and interest in menopause or do I leave with unanswered questions?

If you feel you are not getting the information you need, or you have not found adequate relief from your symptoms, consider finding a clinician with a special interest in menopause. Referrals from a professional organization can be helpful (see box on page 30).

The Menopausal Journey: Your Hormonal Road Map

The experience of menopause is much like a journey, and each woman has her own unique interpretation of the "trip." Knowing what to expect and why, like a road map, can make for a smoother excursion. The remainder of this chapter is designed to arm you with the information to do that.

How you experience menopause is much more than just how

hormonal changes affect your body. Many factors other than hormonal shifts determine your symptoms and the extent to which they disrupt your life.

Consider the information we present in the context of a mind/body approach to health. Think about how your lifestyle and perceptions affect how you feel. We hope you will develop a better understanding of the role of hormones in your health, be better able to assess your individual risk factors, and weigh the impact your lifestyle choices can have on easing perimenopausal symptoms and reducing your risk for disease.

Hot flashes

Lainey began having mild hot flashes when she turned fifty. Initially, they were not really disruptive. However, they gradually began to get more intense. "I would feel an intense heat in my upper body. The sensations bordered on painful, my skin would hurt, and almost instantaneously I would get cold and begin to shiver. I couldn't tell if the temperature was off in the room, or if it was me. It took me a while to figure out that I was waking up several times at night because of these hot flashes. My lack of sleep began to affect me during the day. I felt anxious and I found it hard to make decisions."

If this description sounds familiar, then you understand how months of hot flashes or night sweats can affect all aspects of your life. Hot flashes can be unpredictable, uncomfortable, and embarrassing.

Hot flashes (also known as flushes) are the most common symptom experienced by perimenopausal women in the Western world. A hot flash is classically described as a sensation of sudden, fleeting heat to the chest, face, and head followed by flushing, perspiration, and, sometimes, chills. Palpitations (the sensation of a rapid or irregular heartbeat) and anxiety may also accompany hot flashes. Night sweats are hot flashes that occur during sleep and are accompanied by a drenching sweat. These heat disturbances range enormously in severity and frequency. In fact, the common denominator of the hot flash is how much it can vary from woman to woman. They can be intense and disabling or very mild. Some women experience hot flashes hourly. For others, they are very infrequent.

In the United States, some 25 percent of women seek help for hot flash discomfort and distress during perimenopause. Hot flashes are usually most intense during perimenopause. Some women have hot flashes for a few years, others for only a few months. In rare cases, hot flashes may continue for ten, twenty, or more years after menopause. They tend to be more severe and last longer with surgically induced menopause.

Hot flashes are real; they are not, as some people claim, just "in your head." In fact, during hot flashes, scientists detect increases in heart rate, blood flow, and temperature. Yet scientists do not completely understand the causes. It appears hot flashes are related to falling levels of estrogen during times of hormonal fluctuation. Estrogen plays a role in temperature regulation. Most theories attempting to explain hot flashes involve a dysregulation of the body's tempera-

Culture Flash

Approximately 80 percent of menopausal women in North America and northern Europe notice hot flashes during the menopausal transition. While women in many cultures experience them, the incidence varies. In Japan, only about 25 percent of women report having hot flashes. In fact, there's no expression for a hot flash in the Japanese language. In Mexico, Mayan women from the Yucatan Peninsula do not report having hot flashes. Menstrual irregularity is the only perimenopausal symptom they mention. It is unclear why there is such a discrepancy. Researchers are looking into the role of genetics, lifestyle habits, and even perception, to account for these differences.

ture control, which is set via a complex interaction of hormones. Newer theories suggest there may be differences in each woman's "sweat" thresholds, helping to explain why some women have more problems. It appears that women who are more troubled by hot flashes have a lowered set point at which they sweat, such that a small rise in core body temperature, from a cup of coffee or a hot room, let's say, will cause them to go into a sweat. Robert Freedman, Ph.D., has suggested that these changes may be linked to differences in the activation of stress hormones, which may partly explain why relaxation techniques help. Although we can't explain why and when a hot flash will occur, many women report the following as common "triggers":

- Heat
- Alcohol
- Hot drinks or spicy foods
- Caffeine

Mind/Body Perspectives

Our program helps women pinpoint hot flash triggers. Our experience: Once you begin listening to your body, you have taken the first steps towards cooling off. For example, if you notice a trigger like caffeine or heat, you can avoid those. Emotional triggers like stress or anger are often linked to hot flashes.

If you identify stress as a possible hot flash trigger, consider this: If stress can trigger hot flashes, then it's reasonable that countering your body's reaction to stress or learning skills to better cope with stress will reduce this symptom. That's been our experience and in fact, several studies have demonstrated that eliciting the relaxation response reduces hot flashes. In Chapter 3, we will teach you techniques to do this on your own. In Chapter 8 we offer more specific suggestions for managing hot flashes.

- Some medications (for example, tamoxifen for the treatment of breast cancer and raloxifene for the treatment of osteoporosis)
- Stress

As you can tell, some common triggers are avoidable. Depending on your situation, others may not be. Psychologist Linda Gannon and her colleagues at Southern Illinois University found a strong connection between frequency of hot flashes and stress. Other research suggests that how you perceive hot flashes may influence how you "experience" them. A small mail-in survey in England found that the women who reported more "catastrophic thoughts" about hot flashes also felt the least control over them and most distressed by them. More research is needed to fully understand the causes and effects.

Insomnia, moods, and PMS

Research has yet to sort out the intricate interplay among hormones, mood, sleep, and PMS. Which comes first? The insomnia or the lousy mood? The lousy mood or the PMS? The PMS or the fatigue? If you are perimenopausal and feel irritated, enraged, or exhausted, and suspect hormones are the problem, you join millions of other women. Most are hoping to find a single culprit. But it's just not that simple. Hormones are part of this multidimensional situation, but social and cultural issues are important too. Knowing how each symptom can influence the other is a definite step toward regaining control.

Insomnia and sleep disturbances: Terry began waking up two and three times a night. At the time she had no idea what was wrong. "I didn't understand the physiology of why I was waking up so much or what was happening to my body. I used to be such a sound sleeper." Terry began worrying about not sleeping and not being able to function well the next day. This made the problem worse. She was falling into a vicious cycle. The lack of sleep made it more difficult to deal with hot flashes and other conflicts throughout the day. And she felt a strange restlessness, for which she could not pinpoint a reason. When she finally sought help, she considered herself a wreck.

Insomnia is one of the most common symptoms reported by our patients. Sleep disturbances include difficulty falling asleep, awakening in the middle of the night with difficulty getting back to sleep, and waking early with difficulty getting back to sleep. Chronic poor sleep can undermine your ability to concentrate, make you feel tense and unmotivated, fatigued and irritable, and make it difficult to perform once-routine tasks.

Although sleep disturbances have been linked to changing estrogen levels, insomnia that begins about the time of perimenopause may have as much to do with life's stresses as with menopause itself. One study of 135 women, aged thirty-seven to fifty-nine, showed that psychological distress was more closely related to poor sleep patterns than was menopausal status. Conflicts with adolescents, financial problems, young adults returning or remaining at home, divorce, widowhood, aging parents, or a parent's death may all contribute to increased midlife stress. In Terry's case, there were likely a number of factors contributing to her inability to sleep soundly. In addition to the impact of hot flashes, she was dealing with the death of her mother, she had concerns about not sleeping, and she felt anxious. As you can see, sleep problems can be difficult to sort out.

The role of hot flashes in the insomnia of menopause is complicated, controversial, and not clearly understood. Several studies, which measured sleep patterns, show an association between hot flashes and sleep disruption. If you've ever awoken in a drenching sweat, this isn't news to you. Yet many midlife women report insomnia in the absence of hot flashes. Some evidence suggests that some women wake up due to temperature dysregulation without the perception of a hot flash. While this may factor into some reports of insomnia without hot flash symptoms, the consensus is that there are many other factors.

Not all midlife sleep disturbances are related to menopausal symptoms, stress, or hormone shifts. Rima could not figure out why she felt exhausted. She thought she was sleeping, but her doctor discovered that she had sleep apnea. Her breathing would stop numerous times each night, compromising the quality of her sleep. "It took ten years to be properly diagnosed. I was labeled with everything from chronic fatigue to fibromyalgia. I went through all kinds of specialists. Because of the exhaustion and being run down, mentally I know I was not operating at peak. And I had a lot of health problems, which I think were related to the sleep loss." Treating the sleep apnea lifted her constant state of sleepiness and improved her energy.

Rima's case raises an important point. A number of sleep disorders are more common as we age and they aren't necessarily related to menopause. In addition to sleep apnea (pauses in breathing), women also more frequently experience restless legs syndrome ("creeping" sensations in the lower extremities) and periodic limb movements (limb movements during sleep) after menopause. However, we don't know whether this is related to age in general, the loss of the protective effect of hormones, or other factors.

As we age, our sleep patterns change. Sleep quality declines in midlife for both men and women. We sleep more lightly, and wake up more often and for longer intervals. Aging of the parts of the brain involved in sleep may be part of the cause, as are the many other, previously mentioned and often stressful, life events.

PMS, mood, and attitudes at midlife: If you've ever experienced severe PMS, you know it's a real, biological phenomenon that can throw your body and mind into a state of disarray. PMS-related mood swings appear linked to the effect of wide hormonal fluctuations on the brain's neurotransmitters. Perimenopause is a time of great hormonal flux, so it isn't surprising that it might set the stage for the onset or increase of PMS symptoms. Add in life's stresses and poor sleep quality and you've got a recipe for what has been described as "blue moods."

It's estimated that about 10 percent of women experience mood swings during perimenopause. These changes are temporary for most women. But a history of PMS or postpartum depression appears to increase the likelihood of bothersome symptoms during perimenopause. This suggests that there is a subgroup of women especially vulnerable to mood disturbances at times of hormonal fluctuations. Whatever your experience, it is important to factor in other possible influences. The Melbourne Women's Midlife Health Project offers some insight. Dr. Lorraine Dennerstein at the University of Melbourne led this research, which is one of the few long-term population studies looking at well-being during the menopausal transition. While following midlife women over time, the researchers found that mood (positive or negative) did not seem to correspond to any of the hormones they measured. (Keep in mind, however, that it is difficult to characterize changes in hormonal levels during the menopausal transition.) What they did find, however, was that during the menopausal transition, women are more vulnerable to stressors.

It may be impossible to completely sort out sleep issues, sensitivity to hormones, and sensitivity to life's stresses. But figuring out what may be contributing factors is definitely worth doing. Once you identify the underlying issues, it will be easier to find solutions.

It has been a common (mis)assumption, even among health care providers, that menopause causes depression. One participant in our program revealed that her mother had committed suicide when she turned fifty. The woman's immediate conclusion was that she, too, would succumb to a deep depression when she reached menopause. But studies show menopause does not cause depression. Depression

Perimenopause Does Not Equal Clinical Depression

There is a difference between the mood swings related to perimenopause and depression. Clinical depression is a serious illness, requires treatment, and is twice as common in women as it is in men. Research has shown that a combination of medication and psychotherapy is the most effective treatment.

If you have ever had a major depression, you will recognize its hallmarks. Work, school, relationships, and other aspects of your life may be derailed or put on hold indefinitely. You feel constantly sad or burdened, or you lose interest in all activities, even those you previously enjoyed. This holds true nearly all day, on most days, and lasts at least two weeks. During this time, you also experience at least four of the following signs of depression:

- A change in appetite that sometimes leads to weight loss or gain
- Insomnia or, less often, oversleeping
- A slowdown in talking and performing other tasks or, conversely, restlessness and an inability to sit still
- Loss of energy or feeling tired much of the time
- Feelings of worthlessness or excessive, inappropriate guilt
- Problems concentrating or making decisions
- Thoughts of death or suicide, or suicide plans or attempts

Other signs can include a loss of sexual desire, pessimistic or hopeless feelings, and physical symptoms such as headaches, unexplained aches and pains, or digestive problems.

If you fit the criteria above, call your clinician. There are effective treatments that can greatly relieve symptoms.

in women has been found to peak in their thirties, not their forties. In reality, rates of depression decline after menopause.

The Melbourne Women's Midlife Health Project found no increase in the incidence of major depression or negative moods with menopause. They reported that despite life's stresses and menopausal symptoms, many women at midlife were more likely to report positive moods than negative moods.

Work by Dr. Nancy Woods and the Seattle Midlife Women's Health Study has also helped debunk the idea that waning estrogen makes women inherently depressed. Here, study investigators followed 205 women as they passed through the menopause transition. They found no significant association between depressed mood, menopause, hormone levels, or age. Their research suggested that a woman's outlook actually improved as she passed through the transition. The factors that most accurately predicted feelings of well-being tended to be some of the very topics we address in our mind/body programs. They included:

Mind/Body Perspectives

Many of the factors linked with emotional well-being during midlife lie within your control. They have to do with how you handle life stressors and what you can do to maintain good health. This broader context includes your perceptions, relationships, support networks, and lifestyle.

It is clear that insomnia, mood, and PMS are related. Often patients who reconstruct or change negative thought patterns can ease all three symptoms. Data from our programs and studies show that a mind/body approach that includes lifestyle behaviors, cognitive work, and regular practice of the relaxation response can effectively improve sleep. In studies conducted by Dr. Gregg Jacobs, 100 percent of study participants reported improved sleep. (See Chapter 8.) Regular practice of the relaxation response alone can decrease severity of PMS symptoms. In studies conducted by Dr. Alice Domar, study participants reported symptoms decreased by 58 percent. We've had similar successes in reducing anxiety and depressive symptoms. The mind is a powerful tool. (We give you the skills to harness its power beginning in Chapter 3.)

- good health
- adequate income
- social support
- positive perceptions of stress and health

Women with severe and extended menopausal symptoms do experience negative moods. The Melbourne Women's Midlife Health Project reported that women undergoing surgical menopause (in which symptoms tend to be more severe) and women who had menstrual problems before menopause reported more negative feelings. The study showed that other contributors to negative mood included prior depression, health issues, negative attitudes about menopause, and social and family stressors.

Memory and cognition

Many women in our programs raise concerns about memory lapses, "fuzzy thinking," and problems with concentration. Claire began to worry when she couldn't seem to remember names. "I would just have a lapse, then remember out of the clear blue about a half hour later," she recalls. For Sheila, the problem was a lack of concentration.

Women at and around menopause do worry about the significance of short-term memory problems and difficulty concentrating. Media reports linking estrogen and Alzheimer's disease have likely sharpened these fears. Before you panic over misplaced names and incomplete grocery lists, let's set the record straight about the aging brain.

As we get older, both men and women experience some memory loss. Long-term memory remains better than short-term memory. This is why it can be hard to remember the name of someone you just met, while the name of the ice cream man you knew as a ten-year-old is clear as a bell. Genetics, aging, lifestyle, social status, stress, and sleep are all thought to factor into our cognitive abilities. At this point, there is no clear evidence that links menopause to memory loss. Still, hormone levels do affect our minds as well as our bodies.

What about estrogen specifically? The simple answer is that we don't know. The brain, like other areas of the body, has estrogen receptors; so, estrogen does affect neurotransmitter systems. Animal studies have shown that estrogen has beneficial effects in parts of the brain that govern learning and memory. However, estrogen's role in protecting against Alzheimer's disease remains controversial (see Chapter 9). Estrogen isn't the only relevant hormone. Other hormones such as progesterone and androgens also play a role in maintaining brain function. Genetics is likely another contributor. Other factors believed to increase risk include high blood pressure, high cholesterol, and prior head trauma.

A true understanding of midlife memory concerns is more complex than a simple link to the hormone estrogen. Observations from the Seattle Midlife Women's Health Study encourage a wider lens. Its data suggest that a woman's perception of her memory is more closely related to her perceptions of her health, the presence of a depressed mood, and whether or not she feels stressed than to either menopausal stage or age.

You may be surprised and relieved to learn that stress can biologically impact memory. When we are stressed, our central nervous sys-

Mind/Body Perspectives

Worried about your memory? Review your lifestyle. Are you sleeping well, eating right, and taking care of yourself? Are you overworked or overtired? Keep in mind that poor sleep, often caused by stress, can impact memory. Think about when you've been forgetful. How often is stress the backdrop? Look at what's going on in your life. There is a good chance you're trying to focus on too many things and taking care of everyone but yourself. A combination of mind/body skills can greatly help.

tem reacts: our brain focuses on the perceived threat and is prevented from concentrating on other tasks at hand. Thus if you are worrying about whether you paid the utility bill, you may have trouble attending to your work because your brain is paying attention to the perceived threat (that your power might get shut off). No wonder concentration is compromised. Learning is blocked, memory becomes imprecise, and we easily overlook details. We tend to turn one thought over and over in our brains. Because we can't get past it, it becomes difficult to process many thoughts at once. This part of our evolutionary heritage has helped to ensure our survival. It does not help, however, in the middle of a busy meeting. Physical and psychological conditions can also trigger memory loss or confusion. Depression, traumatic stress, thyroid dysfunction, and vitamin B_{12} deficiency all can affect memory. It's important to treat any underlying medical conditions, so if you have concerns about your memory, check with your clinician.

Sexuality and urogenital health

Many women who enter our programs have questions or concerns about their sexuality. Some fear they will lose their sex drive or experience changes that will limit a healthy sex life. Women today want to maintain a sense of sexuality long past menopause. If you share these sentiments: good news. Polls show sexuality remains an important form of intimacy into our golden years. An AARP survey published in 1999 found that the greatest predictor of sexual satisfaction in postmenopausal women was the availability of a partner, not the physical changes linked to menopause. The *Modern Maturity* sexuality survey included 1,384 adults ages forty-five and older. About two-thirds described themselves as "extremely" or "very satisfied" with their physical relationships. Most of the men and women polled described their partners as "my best friend."

Dr. Robert Butler, president and CEO of the International Longevity Center and founding director of the National Institute on Aging, frequently addresses the issue of sexuality and aging. According to Butler, "Aging per se does not lead to the cessation of sexual activity. Rather, a variety of medical, psychological, and social obstacles can interfere with the expression of sexuality. Believe it or not, love and sex can be better after age sixty than before." Couples who have built an intimate bond know this.

According to researchers, the contributors to a healthy sex life during midlife are generally not related to menopause, with the exception of vaginal dryness. The primary determinants are a mixture of social, psychological, and medical factors including:

- a woman's premenopausal sexuality
- availability of a partner
- functional capacity of her partner
- a woman's perception of her body
- stress/depression
- concurrent health problems
- medications
- personal and cultural expectations of sexual function

Good health, a loving relationship, an available partner, and positive attitudes about sex are crucial to sexual satisfaction. Of course, physical symptoms related to menopause, like vaginal dryness, also play an important role.

Understanding the physical and emotional changes you might experience as you move through the menopause transition will help you to find solutions. One woman whose sex life came to an end many years ago admitted she had never known that vaginal dryness was related to estrogen levels or that a lubricant could help her overcome the problem. This was not a topic she felt comfortable bringing up to her clinician. Yet, if she had known this, there's a chance she could have enjoyed many more years in an intimate relationship with her husband.

During perimenopause, one of the changes a woman may notice is a decrease in natural lubrication when sexually aroused. Over time, low estrogen levels can lead to a thinning of vaginal tissue and decreased elasticity and blood flow. Other related problems include dryness, itching, and irritation. Any of these can cause discomfort during intercourse. For some women this is temporary. For others it may continue or worsen. When vaginal dryness does occur, it is treatable and not always a problem. Regular sexual activity increases blood and oxygen flow to the tissues, helping to maintain vaginal health. In fact, research shows that women are less likely to experience the effects of midlife vaginal changes if they have regular sexual stimulation, including masturbation.

You may notice it takes longer to get aroused during sexual activity. There are a few physical reasons for this. Ebbing hormones can alter sensory perception, nerve transmission, blood flow, and muscle

Mind/Body Perspectives

Intimacy and comfort with our partner largely determine why, how, and whether we respond in a sexual setting. Learning to express your needs to your partner, exploring new ways of communicating sexually, navigating new areas of the body, and improving intimacy all help to keep sex great at any age. Keep in mind that interpersonal stress and the effect of daily hassles can make menopausal symptoms (e.g., hot flashes, insomnia) worse. This in turn can understandably leave a woman feeling less than interested in sex. Our mind/body toolbox includes many skills for improving your ability to cope with stress along with skills to improve communication and intimacy. Together, they can help to enhance your sense of fulfillment in both your relationships and your sex life.

tension. The result may include decreased sensitivity to touch, and ultimately changes in the ability to become aroused. Arousal still occurs, it just may take longer and there is definitely an emotional link.

The role of desire in sexuality is evident and the basis of countless novels. But we don't really know what's behind it. Sexual desire decreases with age for both men and women. For women, exactly how menopause and hormones may contribute to this change is unknown. Falling estrogen levels are associated with decreases in sexual desire during the menopausal transition. Aging ovaries also produce less androgen (testosterone). Testosterone treatments may enhance sexual desire for some women. But there are still questions about its effectiveness, side effects, and long-term health consequences. It is difficult to objectively measure sexual desire because it is inexplicably connected to our emotions. The chemicals linked to libido are triggered by thoughts, fantasies, and attraction. While our expectations and cultural values concerning sex help guide our actions, it's the psychological and interpersonal aspect that most influences us. This is why some consider the brain the most important "sexual organ."

The goal of this chapter has been to give you a new way of looking at your symptoms. Are you beginning to see the connections between how you feel physically and how you feel emotionally? The rest of this book offers skills and knowledge to put you on the path to managing menopause—mind and body!

CHAPTER 3

The Relaxation Response

When we feel hungry, we eat. When we are thirsty we drink. If we overexert ourselves, we sit down and rest. So why is it that when we are stressed we don't try to do something to relax? In this chapter we look at the biology of stress, how it affects the female body, and how to help ease the symptoms of menopause using a physiological state that is the opposite of stress.

Decades of research demonstrate how chronic stress puts us at risk for disease. We inherently know it's not good for our emotional well-being. But we often don't consider the link between stress and our menstrual cycles, menopausal symptoms, fertility, and sex drive.

Fortunately, we all have an inborn mechanism that can counterbalance the harmful effects of stress on the body. This physiological state is known as the *relaxation response* (RR) and we can elicit it at will to create a state of profound peace and rest. It grows easier with practice, and the results are worth the effort. Practiced on a regular basis, the relaxation response provides a soothing balm to your body, mind, and spirit, and can ease many menopausal symptoms. The relaxation response is so fundamental to wellness that it forms the foundation for all of the programs offered through the Mind/Body Medical Institute, including our menopause program.

The Fight-or-Flight Response

To appreciate the healing power of the relaxation response, you must first understand the stress state called the fight-or-flight response. The fight-or-flight response evolved as a survival mechanism. When our ancient ancestors were confronted with a life-threatening situation (like an approaching tiger), the body automatically shifted into a mode that enabled the person to fight off the threat or flee for his life.

Chances are, you have experienced your own version of an approaching tiger at least once. Perhaps you have stepped off a curb into a street and suddenly heard the screech of tires. Maybe, just for a moment, you lost the grip of a child's hand at a busy intersection. How did you feel during those moments? How did you react? Probably, within seconds, your heart started pounding, your muscles tensed, and without even thinking about it, you acted. Maybe you jumped to avoid an oncoming car. Maybe you plucked a child from the roadway. And these were only the changes you were most aware of. Unbeknownst to you, your blood pressure and metabolism also increased significantly, along with your heart and breathing rates. Without even realizing it, in fight-or-flight mode, our bodies adapt quickly and dramatically.

All of these changes are caused by the activation of the hypothalamus, a nerve center imbedded in the underside of the brain. As discussed in Chapter 2, this is also the part of the brain that controls the release of hormones necessary for reproduction. The hypothalamus serves, in some respects, as a central relay station. Stimulated by the cerebral cortex, it monitors incoming information and orchestrates various physiological responses. When the brain detects a threat, the hypothalamus triggers the release of powerful hormones that mobilize systems that save us (increased heart rate, blood pressure, breathing rate, metabolism, and muscle tension). At the same time, it puts on hold the functions not needed in acute life-threatening situations (such as reproduction, digestion, and growth).

Fortunately in the modern world we don't often encounter physically life-threatening situations like saber-toothed tigers. Instead, we react to tensions at the office, financial worries, traffic jams, crowded lines, or stressed relationships as perceived threats. The problem is, the human brain does not distinguish between a true life-threatening situation and a perceived or believed threat. It reacts to both in the same way. Even thinking about a stressful or threatening situation is enough to trigger the same intensity of response.

What is stress? We define stress as the *perception* of a threat to your physical or psychological well-being and the *perception* that you don't have the skills to cope.

The Biology of Stress

To make it simple: the flight-or-fight response temporarily shuts down activities that can wait a few minutes while you survive a lion attack (or a stalled supermarket line, or a disagreement with your teenager). At the same time it boosts those physiological responses required for survival. For example, like digestion and growth, sex is one of those things that can wait until you're done running for your life. The flood of hormones released in the stress response temporarily shuts down sexual response in both males and females.

Here's how it works. As the hypothalamus takes in information from the outside world, it serves as a command post, issuing instructions and dispatching chemicals. These chemicals ultimately put some systems into "lockdown" mode, while kicking others into "hyperdrive." The hypothalamus delivers instructions via specific neuro-hormones to the nearby pituitary gland, which sends out its own chemical messengers. The endocrine glands (thyroid, parathyroid, adrenals, pancreas, ovaries, and in men, the testes) are instructed to stop or start making hormones. By producing chemical messengers, the endocrine system controls an amazing number of vital functions, from bone density and growth to digestion and reproduction. When the body is in fight-or-flight mode, there are ultimately changes to three major systems: the endocrine, the nervous system, and the body's immune systems. As you might imagine, these systems coordinate numerous other systems and control much of our functioning as human beings. Thus, a change has broad implications.

The race: To understand the cascading "chemical avalanche," imagine the hypothalamus as a starting gate for a relay race that will hit all the major pathways of the body. Upon release from the hypothalamus,

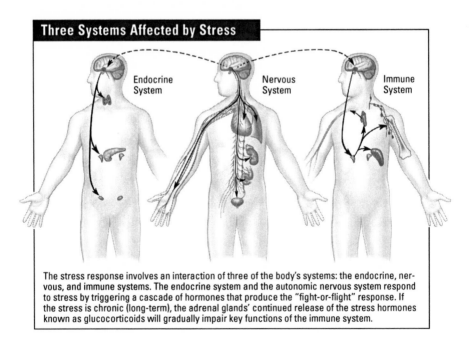

Three Systems Affected by Stress

Endocrine System

Nervous System

Immune System

The stress response involves an interaction of three of the body's systems: the endocrine, nervous, and immune systems. The endocrine system and the autonomic nervous system respond to stress by triggering a cascade of hormones that produce the "fight-or-flight" response. If the stress is chronic (long-term), the adrenal glands' continued release of the stress hormones known as glucocorticoids will gradually impair key functions of the immune system.

chemical messengers speed to deliver news of danger. One of the first of many "handoffs" involves the adrenal glands, which sit atop the kidneys. When they get the signal, the adrenal glands fire off the hormone epinephrine (a.k.a. adrenaline). The hypothalamus then prompts the nerve endings to secrete norepinephrine (a.k.a. noradrenaline). Adrenaline and norepinephrine are key hormones that kick the body into high gear. Heart rate, blood pressure, and the volume of blood being pumped by the heart all increase. Cells respond to

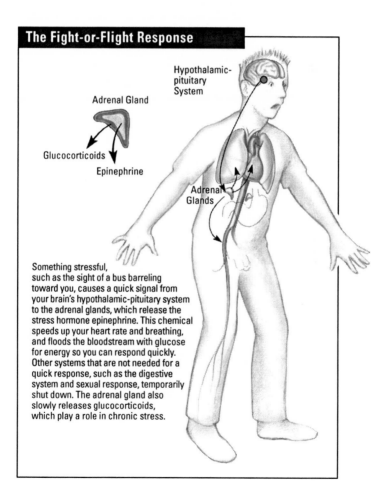

The Fight-or-Flight Response

Hypothalamic-pituitary System

Adrenal Gland

Glucocorticoids

Epinephrine

Adrenal Glands

Something stressful, such as the sight of a bus barreling toward you, causes a quick signal from your brain's hypothalamic-pituitary system to the adrenal glands, which release the stress hormone epinephrine. This chemical speeds up your heart rate and breathing, and floods the bloodstream with glucose for energy so you can respond quickly. Other systems that are not needed for a quick response, such as the digestive system and sexual response, temporarily shut down. The adrenal gland also slowly releases glucocorticoids, which play a role in chronic stress.

these hormonal signals by immediately converting stored glycogen into glucose to boost the body's energy level.

Needless to say, the musculoskeletal system must be activated quickly. To make this efficient, the motor cortex sends signals directly to the muscles when a threat is perceived, increasing tension. As a result, muscles in the jaw, shoulders, and back tighten. You're now physically braced to encounter a threat.

Still other changes affect the immune system. Stress causes the hypothalamus to release a hormone called CRH (corticotropin-releasing hormone). CRH is a principal regulator. It triggers the pituitary gland to release ACTH (adrenocorticotropic hormone), which signals the adrenal glands to secrete the hormones cortisol, corticosterone, and aldosterone. These stress hormones modulate the immune system, ultimately dampening our immunity.

The restraint: Our bodies only have a limited amount of energy to expend, so it makes sense to hold off on nonessential activity when in crisis mode. To conduct this sort of triage, the hypothalamus relies on two major components of the nervous system: the sympathetic nervous system (which tends to speed things up) and the parasympathetic system (which slows them down). As the sympathetic nervous system revs up the body, the parasympathetic nervous system puts the brakes on other systems by unleashing additional hormones that constrict specific blood vessels. This directs blood flow away from nonessential areas (for example, the skin and digestive organs) and directs it to the brain and muscles, which are crucial to a rapid emergency response. The redirection of hormones also slows functions like growth and sex drive.

The results: If you're escaping an oncoming car, the results of the fight-or-flight response are great. You leap to safety. And as you relax the body returns to normal. If, on the other hand, you are plagued with chronic stress, the fight-or-flight response becomes a truly unwelcome "house guest"—one that can have disastrous effects throughout the body. Chronic stress can damage your coronary arteries, throw off your insulin regulation, cause gastrointestinal ailments, and hamper your immune response. For those at risk for heart disease, too much stress can be deadly. The stress response increases blood levels of glucose, cholesterol, and triglycerides, to provide you with energy to fight, while causing blood to clot more quickly in case you are injured. This is exactly the type of blood "profile" that increases the risk of a heart attack.

The list of stress-related ailments is long. As the body temporarily shuts off noncritical processes like growth, hormones inhibit the deposition of calcium in bone, linking stress to bone loss and skeletal atrophy. Stress, as you may have noticed, also doesn't do much for concentration, memory, or relationships with your loved ones. For both emotional and physical reasons, it also can wreak havoc on your sex life, even your menstrual cycles.

Stress and Reproduction

The effects of chronic stress on the reproductive system have been documented throughout history, even as far back as Hippocrates. We know that female athletes who train hard and have little body fat run the chance of a temporary loss of their periods (amenorrhea). Women with eating disorders also are at high risk for amenorrhea. To the body, extreme exercise or lack of food are signs (or cues) that it's not an optimum time to reproduce. As a result of such physical stressors, ovulation can change or cease.

Fascinating research offers some insights into how emotional stress also significantly affects the reproductive cycle. About 5 percent of young women have a condition called stress-induced or hypothalamic amenorrhea. The rate of this condition increases dramatically in proportion to chronic stress, and can reach 100 percent in prisoners before execution. According to researcher Dr. George Chrousos, when severe enough, stress can completely inhibit the female reproductive system. Stress can interfere with the release of luteinizing hormone (LH) and follicle stimulating hormone (FSH), which can affect the release of eggs and ultimately the menstrual cycle. Dr. Sarah Berga, researcher at the University of Pittsburgh, has demonstrated that multiple stressors, such as combining exercise with dietary restriction and social stress, can lead to amenorrhea.

The movement of reproductive hormones is exquisitely complex and not fully understood. Animal studies show certain hormones released in larger amounts during times of stress (CRH, ACTH, cortisol, glucocorticoids, beta-endorphins) can suppress LH, FSH, ovarian estrogen, and progesterone secretion. The various pathways involve the inhibition of gonadotropin-releasing hormone (GnRH). GnRH is released in pulses, with each pulse then prompting the release of LH and FSH at specific times. By interrupting these GnRH pulses, stress hormones can affect reproductive hormones and therefore the reproductive cycle. While there is much to learn about this complex system, stress is frequently linked to both infertility and menopausal symptoms.

The Symptoms of Chronic Stress

Given that activation of these stress pathways triggers profound physiological changes, it is clear that experiencing stress on a regular basis takes a toll. Our bodies just aren't meant to be in a constant state of arousal and fright. You can literally work yourself up into a state of hyperarousal in which your reactions to even the most minor of stresses (like having your teenager look at you the wrong way) become major blowups.

When stress becomes a constant in our lives, there are physical, psychological, and behavioral consequences. Chronic stress exacer-

WARNING SIGNS OF STRESS	
Cognitive Symptoms	**Physiological Symptoms**
• Anxious thoughts	• Stiff or tense muscles
• Fearful anticipation	• Grinding teeth
• Poor concentration	• Sweating
• Memory problems	• Tension headaches
Emotional Symptoms	• Fainting or lightheadedness
	• Choking sensation
• Feelings of tension	• Difficulty in swallowing
• Irritability	• Stomachache
• Restlessness	• Nausea
• Worry	• Vomiting
• Inability to relax	• Loosening of bowels
• Depression	• Constipation
Behavioral Symptoms	• Frequency and urgency of urination
• Avoidance of tasks	• Loss of interest in sex
• Sleep problems	• Tiredness
• Difficulty in completing work assignments	• Shakiness or tremors
• Fidgeting	• Weight loss or gain
• Tremors	• Awareness of heartbeat
• Strained face	**Social Symptoms**
• Fist clenching	• Need to be with others
• Crying	• Social withdrawal
• Changes in drinking, eating, or smoking behaviors	• Deterioration in quality of relationships

bates insomnia, headaches, neck and shoulder pain, hot flashes, and stomach problems, among other things. When you consider the physical changes that are part of the stress response, it is easy to understand why long-term stress can lead to high blood pressure or heart disease and can affect the body's immune system and possibly its susceptibility to various diseases.

Psychologically, when we are chronically stressed we are prone to emotions such as tearfulness, anxiety, depression, anger, and even

PMS. Immersed in stress, we may feel so overwhelmed we can't "think straight." It also affects how we act. (See the stress test in Chapter 1.) Most of us know that when stress levels rise, it is all too easy to fall back on behaviors that we know aren't good for us, but that give us instant gratification. Thus eating disorders, smoking, alcohol and drug abuse are ways in which we often seek to soothe ourselves, but that ultimately impact our health in a negative way.

Such maladaptive coping behavior combined with a lack of self-care can ultimately turn stress into a contributor to long-term illness. We see this in patients with chronic stress-related conditions, who, for lack of psychological care and self-help strategies, never get better. When stress is a factor in ill health—whether the condition is migraines, back pain, PMS, or heart disease—drugs or surgery may be necessary, but they won't be sufficient. Patients continue to suffer with stubborn symptoms and the economic costs are incalculable.

Obviously, it's important to find ways to counteract the stress response so that we don't subject our bodies to all that wear and tear. Fortunately, we possess a natural and innate protective mechanism to do just that: the relaxation response.

The Relaxation Response

The relaxation response is a powerful tool in its ability to make people feel better, and we have found that women dealing with menopausal symptoms are greatly relieved when they begin a regular practice. Lauren, a fifty-year-old banker, arrived at our program feeling as if her life was out of control: "I was having incredible night sweats. I would literally splash. I was exhausted and depressed. I didn't feel sharp or on top of my game. Everything converged. Then I had a mammogram that showed a lump and I had to go for a breast biopsy." Lauren recalls that her hot flashes started getting worse around the time of the breast biopsy. Fortunately, it was benign. But during that week, Lauren began to realize the toll that stress could take on her physical and emotional well-being.

It is no real surprise that women feel better when they quiet their minds and their bodies. For thousands of years, many cultures have incorporated traditions that elicit the relaxation response (RR). This physiological state puts the brakes on the runaway biological changes that first put us into overdrive. Eliciting the RR quiets the sympathetic nervous system. Your heartbeat and breathing return to normal. Oxygen consumption decreases and blood flows more easily throughout your body.

Electrical activity of the brain also changes during the RR. Electroencephalogram (EEG) readings, which record brain wave activity, show the RR increases the frequency and intensity of alpha and theta slow brain waves in the cerebral cortex, the site of higher mental functions. These types of brain waves are associated with a calm yet alert state of mind. This may explain, in part, why women report improved mental clarity in our programs.

Those who regularly elicit the relaxation response enjoy lasting effects that buffer their long-term sensitivity to stress. Faced with a threat, it allows them to experience the same flood of stress hormones

Physiological Changes Compared

	Fight-or-Flight Response	Relaxation Response
Metabolism	Increases	Decreases
Heart rate	Increases	Decreases
Blood pressure	Increases	Decreases
Breathing rate	Increases	Decreases
Muscle tension	Increases	Decreases

Benefits of the Relaxation Response

- Reduction of physical symptoms related to stress
- Less anxiety; greater equanimity
- Less compulsive worrying, negative thinking, and self-criticism
- Better ability to concentrate and greater awareness
- More energy
- Self-acceptance
- Feeling of peace

that we all do, but they don't react as strongly. One researcher, for instance, conducted a study in which he subjected volunteers to stress. He found that people who regularly elicited the relaxation response produced elevated levels of norepinephrine in response to stress, just as other volunteers did, but their blood pressure and heart rate did not increase as much as the others.

After identifying her hot flash triggers, Lauren, who had been dealing with night sweats, fatigue, and mood swings, began slowing down long enough to start a regular RR practice. She started listening to RR tapes and taking short RR breaks during the day: "I can feel my stress disappearing. I use it when I go to bed. I'm no longer stressed about sleeping. I also use it when I'm going into difficult business meetings." Lauren later learned a variety of ways to elicit the relaxation response and how to fit it into her busy schedule, which we'll discuss later in the chapter.

Eliciting the Relaxation Response

You can best call forth the relaxation response simply by *letting go.* This may be hard for the woman juggling many roles. You can't pursue the relaxation response the way that you may pursue other goals in your life, by jumping over a series of hurdles. You must lower barriers rather than jump over them so that, in effect, relaxation comes to you. This is a different way of thinking, but it is well worth the effort and time to learn it.

Attaining the physiological state that is the relaxation response can be brought about in a variety of ways, but all techniques have two basic components. First is the *focusing of attention* through repetition of word, prayer, phrase, or physical activity; and the second is the *passive disregard of everyday thoughts* when they occur, and the return to the repetition. Because eliciting the relaxation response is unique for each person, we teach our patients a variety of techniques, all of which can get you to that place of peace and relaxation. We encourage women to experiment and see which method works best for them. Some women settle on one technique, others approach it the way an athlete approaches cross-training, using different techniques for different situations and moods. In a sense, it's cross-training for the soul.

Quieting the Mind

Passive disregard of everyday thoughts is easier said than done! Negative thoughts can pose a barrier to relaxation. You may find, as many of our patients do, that as soon as you quiet down, your mind begins to race. Remember that negative thoughts can stimulate the stress response. Try to notice your thoughts as they come, and then, without judgment, let them go. It may feel odd at first to *plan* relaxation, but once you sample different methods, find out which ones work best for you, practice them regularly, and begin to feel better, eliciting the relaxation response will be something you look forward to—and a tool you can call upon for the rest of your life.

Techniques to Elicit the Relaxation Response

- Diaphragmatic breathing
- Meditation
- Imagery or visualization
- Yoga
- Body scan
- Progressive muscle relaxation
- Mindfulness
- Autogenic training (suggestive phrases used to bring about self-directed change)
- Practice using repetitive focus (word or cadence)
- Repetitive prayer

The Breath of Life

Life is in the breath. He who half breathes, half lives.

—PROVERB

Breathing is one of the simplest, yet most powerful techniques you can use to elicit the relaxation response. Paced respiration has also been associated with decreasing hot flashes. (See Chapter 8.) The simple act of breathing is so vital to life that it can center us to the moment, an essential component of the relaxation response. Despite its importance, we often don't get the full potential of a good breath. When we're anxious or stressed, there is a natural tendency to hold our breath. So, when tension arises, stop and take a moment to breathe deeply.

Fortunately, breathing is actually one of the few physiological functions that is both voluntary and involuntary in nature. That means we can learn how to modulate our breathing to reduce stress and induce calm. We've found in follow-up surveys that our patients use breathing techniques to deal with stress more consistently than they use other relaxation methods. It may surprise you to learn that there are two distinct ways of breathing, and that one is much more conducive to relaxation than the other.

Women have been conditioned, over the years, to hold in their stomachs for that "flat" tummy. Most of us tend to be chest, or thoracic breathers. If you breathe this way, your shoulders rise and your chest expands as you inhale. Although your lungs do take in air, this is a relatively shallow way of breathing. And if you become tense, angry, or afraid, your breathing tends to quicken, so that your breath comes in short staccato bursts. You may find yourself gasping for breath, and your chest may feel constricted. Breathing this way all the time only fuels anxiety and tension.

A much healthier alternative is diaphragmatic or abdominal

breathing. The diaphragm is a large sheet-like muscle that extends across the bottom of your lungs. It is located above abdominal organs such as the stomach and liver. When you breathe diaphragmatically, your abdomen expands more than your chest. This is the way that we are born breathing, but most of us switch to chest breathing by the time we are adults.

Learning Diaphragmatic Breathing

Diaphragmatic breathing has long been a staple of relaxation techniques and eastern religions. For thousands of years, this deep breathing technique has been used to reduce stress, calm the spirit, and quiet the mind.

The diaphragm adds muscle, literally, to each breath, making each one more powerful. When we breathe in, the diaphragm contracts, so that more air is drawn into the lungs. When we exhale, the diaphragm relaxes and more air exits the lungs. Each breath draws in more life-sustaining oxygen, which helps to produce energy. As air is exhaled, we expel carbon dioxide wastes. By using our diaphragms to help us breathe, we get more benefit from each breath.

Try this exercise to become more aware of the way you breathe now, and gradually shift to diaphragmatic breathing.

1. Lie down on the floor if that's comfortable, or sit in a chair with your buttocks near the edge of the seat while keeping your back straight.
2. Place one hand on your chest and the other on your abdomen, just above your belly button. Take a deep breath. Your lower hand should move more than the one on your chest. Concentrate on drawing air down into your abdomen until your belly rises and falls with each breath.

3. Breathe through your nose rather than your mouth; this will warm the breath, filter air, and enable you to breathe more deeply.

If you have trouble at first, don't worry. As long as you're breathing you're headed in the right direction. It sometimes helps to lie on your back and put an object (like a Walkman or stuffed animal) on your stomach and watch it rise and fall with the breaths. Another technique is to imagine that you are blowing out a candle. Inhale deeply and then exhale with your mouth open slightly and lips rounded. Feel free to make noise as you exhale, either by blowing out air or by sighing as you release it. Focusing on your breathing for ten to fifteen minutes will serve as a breath-focused RR.

Meditation

The word meditation may bring to mind an image of a Hindu priest sitting cross-legged on a cushion. That is one way to meditate, but there are others. We can all meditate, no matter what our culture. It is simply a matter of using the repetition of a "focus" word or phrase to turn our attention inward, rather than paying attention to our thoughts or what is going on in the world around us. Try the following brief practice in meditation:

1. Assume a comfortable position.
2. Take a few deep diaphragmatic breaths to calm your mind and body.
3. Concentrate on a word (or any other mental focus, such as a sound, phrase, or prayer, that you repeat silently to yourself in rhythm with your breath). For example: repeat "I am at peace," "I can relax," or whatever words help you let go and

Breath-Focused Relaxation Response

This breath-focused relaxation response is based on diaphragmatic breathing and involves using a full yogic breath. Although the full yogic breath is one long breath, it is easiest to learn by dividing it into three different phases according to the parts of the body where it is experienced: the abdomen, rib cage, and upper chest. Once you get the hang of it, this is one of the most effective ways to ground yourself in the present and decrease tension and anxiety.

1. Lie on your back on the floor, or find a comfortable seated position. Close your eyes and simply take note of how you are breathing.

2. Now inhale into your belly, causing your abdomen to rise. This brings air deeply into the lower lobes of your lungs. On the out-breath, your abdomen settles back toward the spine. Continue for a few moments observing the breath as the belly rises with each in-breath and falls with each out-breath. You may begin to notice that your breathing rate is becoming slower and the pauses between the breaths are becoming a little longer.

3. Next, see if you can deepen your relaxation by bringing awareness up to your rib cage in the following way: Inhale into your belly as far as it will comfortably expand; then allow yourself to let in a little more air. Notice how the ribs are affected, moving up and out, expanding to either side. Exhale deeply, and watch them fall. Continue in this way, inviting the breath in, first to your belly

bring you feelings of peacefulness, calm, and safety. Religious or spiritual phrases also work well. In the practice of Transcendental Meditation, these are known as "mantras."

4. If your own thoughts or something from the outside world distracts you, take a deep breath and return to your mental focus. Instead of getting caught up in an internal dialogue, gently redirect your attention to your out-breath or your focus

as far as it will comfortably expand, and then up to your rib cage. Exhale and allow for a pause.

4. Now take your breath awareness one step further. Breathe into your belly, then your ribs, and, finally, invite the air into and become aware of your upper chest, noticing how your collarbone lifts ever so slightly, opening the upper lungs. As you exhale fully, see if you can maintain the open and lifted stance of the upper chest as the air moves back and forth.

5. For the next ten to fifteen minutes, practice linking all three phases (belly, ribs, upper chest) of this full yogic breath. Develop a smooth, steady rhythm. Rest in the pause at the end of each out-breath until the in-breath is ready to begin on its own. Some people find it helpful to count. For example, try counting to yourself from one to five as you breathe in. Hold for two additional counts. Then slowly breathe out, counting to five as you do so. Experiment to find your natural rate. You may prefer to connect the qualities of calmness and peacefulness to the breath by repeating silently to yourself on the in-breath: "breathing in peace and calm," and on the out-breath: "breathing out tension and anxiety."

word or phrase. You will find that, with time and practice, this becomes easier.

5. Continue for ten to twenty minutes. (Place a clock nearby, so that when you feel your time is up you can take a quick look and then choose to continue or stop.)

6. Take a few slow deep breaths, stretch, and slowly open your eyes.

Focus Words and Phrases

Listed below are sample words you can use to focus your mind. We encourage you to think of others. The idea is to find words that convey feelings of peace, safety, and acceptance.

Neutral	Spiritual
Calm	Hail Mary
Let go	Lord, have mercy
My time	Our Father, who art in heaven
Ocean	The Lord is my shepherd
One	Echod ("One")
I am at peace	Shalom ("Peace")
I can relax	Sh'ma Yisroel ("Hear, o Israel")
	Om (the universal sound)
	Shantih ("Peace")
	Abba ("Father")
	Maranatha ("Come, Lord")
	Allah

Words to avoid

Words that sound like commands or are normally used in expressing harsh emotions do not make good focus words. Choose words like these, and you may find your blood pressure rising, not falling.

Go

Hurry

Now

Stop

Imagery and Visualization

Imagery has long been the basis for healing rituals in cultures worldwide. Native Americans have summoned images to guide them and vision quests have served to bring meaning and purpose to lives. As the Buddha observed: "We are what we think." But, science has recently begun to prove that visual imagery is not just a phenomenon of the mind. It is also a powerful tool for affecting the body. Images affect us physically and emotionally. Our minds react to a mental image in the same way as they would to a physical object or event.

Harnessing the power of visualization is a great way to elicit the relaxation response and change your mood. We use a number of guided imagery scenarios in our menopause program. Some provide a "cooling" mountain spring for those seeking relief from hot flashes. Others summon images of walks on the beach or floating through the air. All involve picturing a peaceful or comforting setting, focusing your mind on it as it unfolds, and allowing all of your senses to be present to your experience. Sometimes people can do this on their own, as when they think about taking a walk on the beach. Others find it helpful to listen to a tape. (For more information, see the resources section at the end of this book.) Another option is to record these scenarios on tape and play them back whenever you choose.

Try the short visualization exercise that follows, one of the most popular in the menopause program. As with all imagery-based RRs, if the image creates any feelings of stress or anxiety, feel free to alter it in any way so that it works for you.

1. Assume a comfortable position.
2. Close your eyes and take a few deep diaphragmatic breaths. Breathe in a feeling of peace and relaxation, and breathe out tension and stress. Don't force your breath, just notice the rhythm of your breathing.
3. Now imagine yourself standing at the edge of a beautiful meadow. Let all of your senses become aware of your surroundings. What time of the year is it? What time of day? As you walk through the meadow, what do you see? Flowers, birds, insects, colors? What do you hear? Birds, the wind?

What do you smell? The earth? Flowers? What do you feel? The temperature, the wind?

4. You notice that in the middle of the meadow is a beautiful hot air balloon. Look at the pleasing pattern of colors. As you walk up to it, you realize that it is available for you to ride in.

5. As you step into the basket you notice that on the floor are sandbags. Each sandbag has writing on it. As you look closer, you realize that each sandbag represents some burden, stress, or concern in your life.

6. Choose a burden you want to let go of, pick up the appropriate sandbag and let go of it over the side. As you do so the balloon gets lighter, and you notice that with each burden you let go of, you also start to feel lighter. Let go of as many sandbags as you wish.

7. As the balloon gets lighter, so do you; you begin to feel more relaxed and your mind becomes quiet. You float quietly among the clouds, drifting along, feeling content, peaceful, and free of concerns, and enjoying this time of being quiet with yourself.

8. Keep this image and take quiet time for several minutes.

9. It is time to begin your journey back. But remember this is a special balloon and you don't have to pick up your burdens to return to ground.

10. The balloon slowly and gently returns to the meadow. As you return, remember how it felt to let go of certain burdens and concerns so you can repeat the experience when you feel burdened by these stressors in your everyday life.

11. Gently step out of the balloon and begin to walk back through the meadow, again paying attention to the scene around you, focusing on the experience of the moment.

12. As you reach the edge of the meadow, transition back into the room, opening your awareness to this environment.

13. Open your eyes, slowly stretch and begin to move, take deep breaths, yawn, and connect with the energy around you.

Body Scan

When was the last time you paid attention to each part of your body? Often we notice body parts only when they hurt. It turns out we hold stress in many areas of the body, yet we don't even realize it—the jaw, scalp, throat, hands. The goal of the body scan is to become aware of your body and to relax in the process. If you come across tension, use breathing techniques to gradually let it go. This technique helps you to focus on one part of your body at a time, releasing any tension you feel there. You can practice a body scan using the steps below.

1. Start by lying in a comfortable position. Take a few deep diaphragmatic breaths to quiet your mind and body. Close your eyes.
2. Bring your awareness to your right big toe. Think of your toe as being made of atoms, with space between the atoms, so that the toe feels open and spacious.
3. Now bring your awareness to your second, third, fourth, and fifth toes, the ball of your foot, the arch, top of your foot, and allow the whole right foot to relax into the support of the floor, feeling spacious and light.
4. Repeat steps 2 and 3 with your left foot.
5. Next bring your awareness to your right ankle, calf, knee, thigh, and hip. Allow your whole right leg to relax into the support of the floor, feeling open, spacious, and light.
6. Repeat step 5 with your left leg.
7. Now bring your awareness to your buttocks, lower back, middle back, upper back, and notice each vertebra one at a

time, seeing the space around the vertebra as open and spacious, relaxing all the muscles in your back.

8. Bring your awareness now to your abdomen and your chest, and focus on the space inside your lungs as you inhale and exhale, relieving any restrictions that might be there. Allow your whole chest cavity to relax and feel spacious and light and open.

9. Bring your awareness to your right thumb, second, third, fourth, and fifth fingers, the palm of your hand, your wrist, forearm, elbow, upper arm, and shoulder. Feel your whole right arm relax, open, spacious, and light.

10. Repeat step 9 with your left hand and arm.

11. Now bring your awareness to your neck and jaw. Allow your jaw to relax, letting your mouth relax into a gentle smile, an inner smile. Imagine the inside of your throat is spacious. Become aware of your cheeks, your eyes, and allow the eyes to rest in their sockets. Then shift attention to your forehead, softening the muscles. Bring awareness to the top of your head, the back of your head, and your entire scalp.

12. Let your whole body rest softly into the support of the floor. Bring your awareness to your breath. As you inhale, imagine bringing energy and light into your body, and as you exhale, release any tension you may still hold in your body.

13. If you notice that any part of your body is still tense, focus your breath in that area, releasing tension each time you exhale. If your mind wanders, simply acknowledge the thoughts and gently return to your focus or your out-breath.

14. Take a few minutes to notice the experience of yourself when your mind is quiet and your body relaxed.

15. Now it's time to bring your awareness back to the room. Take a few slow deep breaths. Slowly open your eyes. Stretch and yawn if you want.

Progressive Muscle Relaxation

Progressive muscle relaxation is similar to a body scan. But it adds a key variation, the actual tightening of muscles. This is great for people who have difficulty relaxing, or need a more physical way of eliciting the relaxation response. Instead of simply using mental focus and breathing to relax tense muscle groups, this technique requires a conscious increase in tension before letting go. The idea is to tense and then release large muscle groups, such as your shoulders, biceps, and thighs, in a progressive fashion. You might start at the top of your body and work your way downward, or vice versa. Not only does this help you to relax, by releasing the muscle tension, but it also reminds you that you are in control of the tension. And as you relax physically, you will find that you also relax mentally and emotionally. Try this short exercise in progressive muscle relaxation.

1. Sit quietly in a comfortable position in a quiet place.
2. Close your eyes.
3. Begin the muscle relaxation sequence starting with your feet. Stretch your right leg in front of you. Pull the foot back, bringing the toes toward the knee. Feel what the tension is like and where the sensation is felt. Now take a deep breath in, and on the out-breath release all of the tension in the right lower leg and foot. Repeat with the left. The goal is to feel the tension, isolate the sensation, take a deep breath in, and release the tension on the out-breath. Continue this four-step, right-to-left approach for the different muscle groups in this exercise.
4. Tense the muscles of the right thigh as if you are trying to lift your leg against a weight. Repeat with the left thigh.
5. Pinch the buttocks in and up, making them hard. It is as if you were seated upon a rock.
6. Pull the abdomen in, hardening it.

7. Make a fist with your right hand. Repeat with your left.

8. Raise your shoulders up to your ears, the neck disappearing like that of a turtle.

9. Smile, pulling back the corners of your mouth and baring your teeth.

10. Raise your eyebrows and pinch them together.

11. Once you finish tightening and releasing all the muscle groups, do a mental scan of your entire body, from your head down to your toes. If you notice any remaining areas of tension, repeat the tension and release cycle.

12. Now take five deep breaths through your nose, breathing in as slowly as you can, and breathing out as slowly as you can. Then, let the breath come on its own; watch the breath coming in and going out.

13. If you wish, you may continue doing a breath-focused relaxation for ten to twenty minutes. When you finish, stay quiet for several minutes, at first with eyes closed and then with eyes open, allowing yourself to adjust to your surroundings.

Autogenic Training

If you have trouble quieting "mind" chatter, autogenic training may be a good option. Whether this is a problem for you or not, this technique is very effective. It is called "autogenic" because it assists you in self-directed change. The technique is a subtle form of self-hypnosis that helps you bypass your conscious mind in order to instruct your body to relax. Autogenic training uses repetitive phrases about the desired state of the body to induce relaxation. Try this exercise to understand how autogenic training works. If you are having trouble with hot flashes, substitute the word "relaxation" or "calm" for warmth.

1. Find a comfortable place and take a few slow, deep cleansing breaths.
2. Slowly and silently repeat the following phrases to yourself (repeat each phrase two to four times, pausing a few seconds between each repetition).

I am beginning to feel quite quiet.

I am beginning to feel relaxed.

My feet, knees, and hips feel heavy.

Heaviness and warmth are flowing through my feet and legs.

My hands, arms, and shoulders feel heavy.

Warmth and heaviness are flowing through my hands and arms.

My neck, jaw, tongue, and forehead feel relaxed and smooth.

My whole body feels quiet, heavy, and comfortable. I am relaxed.

Warmth and heaviness flow into my arms, hands, and fingertips.

My breathing is slow and regular. I am aware of my calm, regular heartbeat.

My mind is becoming quieter as I focus inward. I feel still.

Deep in my mind I experience myself as relaxed, comfortable, and still. I am alert in a quiet, inward way.

3. Now finish your relaxation and begin to take several deep diaphragmatic breaths as you say the following phrases to yourself: "As I finish my relaxation, I take in several deep, reenergizing breaths, bringing light and energy into every cell of my body."

Whether you prefer autogenic training or imagery, you can mix and match a variety of techniques during your twenty minutes of relaxation response practice. For example, start with a breath focus and move to a body scan followed by an imagery-based RR. Or, begin with a progressive muscle relaxation and then move to an imagery or focus word. As you try different methods, you will likely settle on a few that you really like.

Mindfulness

You've heard the expression, "Stop and smell the roses." Well, if you actually do stop to breathe deeply the scent of a rose, then you've participated in a form of mindfulness. Rooted in the ancient principles of Tibetan Buddhism, mindfulness is both a meditation and a philosophy.

During a normal day, it is common to feel distracted and fragmented, as though your mind is going in ten different directions. Ever open the refrigerator looking for something but can't remember what? Or drive clear past your exit on the highway without noticing? Mindfulness is an antidote for this. It simply asks us to turn our attention to the present moment, which is difficult for most people. How many times have you found your mind running at full speed conjuring up worst-case scenarios or replaying old conflicts? Mindfulness allows us to release the past and stop moving our energies into the future. Mindfulness is a powerful tool in managing emotions like regret, worry, and anxiety. It involves paying attention to what is occurring directly within our field of experience from moment to moment.

Practiced daily, mindfulness grounds us in the present. This means that you are not reliving with regret something that already happened, or anticipating or worrying about something that has not yet happened. Mindfulness is the only method for eliciting the relaxation response that is practiced "in real time"—that is, you don't have to stop to do it! Thus, it is a handy technique if you feel as though you are so busy you can't find fifteen or twenty minutes in your day to meditate. You can use mindfulness when sitting quietly or engaged in various day-to-day activities. Maintain full awareness from moment to moment; focus on one task at a time, and try to really appreciate all aspects of that task. It may help to pick a task you normally consider boring, such as washing the dishes, folding laundry, or weeding the garden. You can focus on the ingredients as you cook dinner, or the motion your body makes as you walk or dance. Be aware of everything you see, hear, smell, touch, and taste during the activity. In other words, be open to the full sensory experience of it, "wake up" to it. Notice what you learn about yourself in the process.

Becoming Mindful

If you're used to whizzing through your day, mindfulness may take some practice. Next time you see a gorgeous sunset, sunlight on leaves, water trickling into a pond, or any image that strikes you as captivating, stop. At this point, allow yourself to truly experience the moment:

1. What colors do you see? Notice different shades, sharp contrasts, or subtle tones. If it's an object, how does it blend into its surroundings?
2. Be aware of any aromas. As you breathe deeply, use your sense of smell.
3. If you can touch it, what is the texture? If you're looking at scenery, do you feel a breeze or the sun on your face?
4. Do you hear any sounds? Are there birds chirping? Is the wind blowing?
5. Before you walk away, contemplate the object or vista, taking in the experience as a whole.
6. When you have finished, notice how you are feeling. Do you feel more grounded or peaceful?

When we become aware of the small things in life, we deepen our appreciation for all that surrounds us. And don't stop with captivating sights and sounds. Begin to notice the everyday faces of people, the tastes of food, and the sounds of life. As you take in the beauty of the world that surrounds you, you will be on your way to living mindfully!

You may begin to realize how much you miss in your everyday life when you are not practicing mindfulness—the taste of your food, the sky at sunset as you walk to your car after work, the spring flowers budding along your front path as you leave for work in the morning.

Yoga

Your body is your teacher, listen to your body's wisdom.

—UNKNOWN

For more than three thousand years, people have relied on the healing power of yoga. Based on Indian philosophical teachings, this ancient practice is a blend of postures, meditation, and deep breathing. And for so many women, it is an essential tool in managing menopausal symptoms.

Women entering our programs often feel disconnected from their bodies. They keep busy schedules and are masters at keeping things together intellectually. Yet, they have become accustomed to ignoring their bodies. The word yoga means "union" or "joining together." For women it is a wonderful way to reconnect with the body while improving balance, increasing vitality, and gaining a sense of empowerment. It can also improve mood.

Ellen, a busy professional who keeps a hectic schedule, tried yoga a few years ago and has since made it a daily ritual. "Yoga is my meditation practice. It's the one thing I can do that takes a hundred percent of my mind." Because her job involves sitting at a computer all day, she prefers this form of moving meditation: "I'm certainly more flexible and stronger and it completely clears the mind."

Yoga postures offer a physical, emotional, and spiritual release. Once you begin practicing yoga on a regular basis, you will learn more about your body because you will be taking the time to listen.

As you do so, you also reap other rewards. Studies show that regular yoga practice improves circulation, digestion, respiration, immune system function, and increases flexibility and muscle tone. As a tool for the mind, it serves as a great way to elicit the relaxation response. And research has shown that daily elicitation of the relaxation response can reduce both intensity and frequency of hot flashes and symptoms of PMS.

There are many types of yoga. Some are actually quite intense, even difficult. To best elicit the relaxation response, we advise trying a gentle form. Certain types of "hatha" yoga are gentle. This is the form we use in our programs. It involves coordinating movement with breathing while moving in and out of postures (or *asanas*). We find it helps to release tension and provides a focus that deepens relaxation.

Every woman's body is unique. So, it's best if yoga is individualized. Therefore we won't try to teach yoga in this book. If you're a beginner, try a class. Many yoga teachers have a special interest in menopause and can teach postures that may help alleviate menopause symptoms. We recommend you seek out an instructor with expertise in this area and inquire beforehand about what you can expect from the class. Once you have learned the basic moves, you may enjoy doing yoga on your own with the help of tapes and books. Because classes offer camaraderie and are relaxing, the best option may be to combine the two.

If you take a class, do ask about tailoring the postures to meet your needs. For example, some women find forward bends are effective in relieving hot flashes, whereas others find that this posture can exacerbate the hot flashes. This is why it's good to try an individualized approach. It can make your yoga experience all the more fulfilling and effective. The ultimate goal is to learn to listen to the wisdom of your body. Try it and notice how great you feel afterward!

"Mini" Relaxation Responses

Minis are like booster shots for the soul. They are miniature versions of techniques used to elicit the relaxation response, and generally take only a minute or so to do. Minis can involve taking a few deep diaphragmatic breaths or doing gentle stretches to relieve tension. They help you stay in the present and extend the benefits of the relaxation response throughout the day. They are quick, powerful, and effective and our patients love them. They are even effective for hot flashes. The beauty of a mini is that it invokes a sense of immediate calm. Some women in our programs report using them as often as one hundred times a day on a bad day.

You can do minis any time and in virtually any location: your car while stuck in traffic, waiting for the bus, at the office, or stuck in the slow line at the supermarket, even during an argument. You can also use minis to deal with situations that many people find stressful: a public speaking event, a visit to the dentist's office, a pelvic exam, a mammogram, or other experiences that cause you fear or anxiety. One of our patients cured her needle phobia by using minis.

Recall Lauren, the busy banker. She has begun to rely on minis to get through stressful periods: "It's like a little secret I carry in my pocket. Minis were like a transformation for me. Before, I would think oh no, I can't handle this. Now I know I can breathe and I imagine myself at the shore taking a walk early in the morning trying to bear in mind the waves and the ocean—and I can feel my stress disappearing." Minis are generally done with your eyes open. Remember, a mini can be as simple as taking one deep diaphragmatic breath.

Mini Version 1

Count very slowly to yourself from ten down to zero, one number for each breath. Thus, with the first diaphragmatic breath, you say "ten" silently to yourself, with the next breath, you say "nine," etc. If you start feeling light-headed or dizzy, slow down the counting, pausing in between the breaths. When you get to "zero," see how you are feeling. If you are feeling better, great. If not, try doing it again. This one is terrific for road rage.

Mini Version 2

Breathe deeply and slowly. As you inhale, silently count from one to five. Then as you exhale, count backwards (five, four, three, two, one). Repeat several times. The counting will help you to slow your breathing and focus your mind. See Chapter 8 for more about the effectiveness of this mini—also called "paced respiration"—for hot flashes.

Mini Version 3

After each inhalation, pause for a few seconds, counting 1, 2, 3. After you exhale, pause again for a few seconds counting 1, 2, 3. Do this for several breaths, resting in the peacefulness of the pauses between the breaths.

Mini Version 4

Coordinate your breath with empowering or soothing messages such as: "I am . . ." (with the in-breath) ". . . at peace" (with the out-breath), or "positive power . . ." (with the in-breath) ". . . negative nonsense" (with the out-breath).

Mini Version 5

Mini stretching: As you breathe in, slowly bring your arms up above your head. Notice the stretch along your sides. Now, put the backs of your hands together and as you breathe out, slowly lower your arms (elbows straight) back down to your sides, as though they were sinking through a vat of warm honey.

Blue dot reminders: Some of our patients find it helpful to use the "blue dot" method to remind themselves to do minis throughout the day. You can buy small adhesive dots in any office supply store. We like blue because it's a restful color. Place the dots on various items in your home or office to remind yourself to do a mini. Many people stick dots on the phone, which can be a source of stress, or on the refrigerator if they tend to be emotional eaters. If one of your stressors is traffic, place a dot on your dashboard.

Minis are great in time of need, as an added tool for relaxation, but they do not replace the benefits of a full relaxation response.

Making the Relaxation Response Work!

If your days are filled with appointments, meetings, or child care, it may be difficult to find the time to get started. But remember, eliciting the relaxation response can help you deal with stress. So, it's a good investment. The following general guidelines will help you make your relaxation experience effective, no matter which method (or combination of methods) you choose.

Choose a time for relaxation: Beginning the morning with a relaxation response technique can be a great way to prepare for the day. This starts the day by quieting your mind and body, so that you are less reactive to the stresses and hassles you will undoubtedly encounter. Many people find it ideal to spend fifteen minutes practicing before breakfast, before the rest of the household is up. But mornings are definitely not the only time when relaxation is good. Some women elicit the relaxation response when they get home from work to clear their minds and reenergize. Whether morning, noon, or night, what's important is that you pick the best time for you.

Find a peaceful place: Find or create a special place where you can elicit the relaxation response without worrying about being interrupted by a ringing telephone, the sounds of the television, pets or family members running in and out. Once you identify a spot that works for you, try to return to the same area every day. As you associate your special place with relaxation, and you give yourself permission to yield to the process, you may find that just returning to it every day will help you to calm down.

Get comfortable: You can elicit the relaxation response in any position that makes you comfortable, as long as it isn't so relaxing that you fall asleep. Most people prefer to sit in a well-padded chair. You can also sit on a big floor pillow or lie down on your back.

Practice regularly: To obtain the most benefit from the relaxation response, elicit it regularly. We recommend practicing once a day for fifteen to twenty minutes, or twice a day for ten minutes at a time. In this way, you attune your body to becoming relaxed, and regularly provide a buffer against the stress hormones circulating in your bloodstream. After about two weeks you may begin to notice this "carryover" effect. Our patients describe a sense of rolling with the punches; things that used to really set them off no longer do. Your body will begin to sense when the time is up, but it is fine to simply open your eyes and check a watch or clock.

Focus, focus, focus: Focusing your mind is a continuous process. If you are like most people, you will find it hard at first to quiet your mind's internal dialogue and random thoughts. As soon as you quiet down, it may seem as if your brain fills with static. That's why all of the relaxation response techniques involve some type of repetitive focus, the breath, a sound, word, or phrase repeated silently or aloud.

Of course, most people who are new to the relaxation response find that their minds do not switch off easily. You may be distracted by thoughts that seem to bubble up from nowhere. This is natural. Your mind was meant to think! The challenge is to let the thoughts come, and then let them go. Don't dwell on them. That is where our last general guideline, a passive attitude, comes in.

A passive attitude: A passive mental attitude is accepting, not judgmental. So as you elicit the relaxation response, try not to evaluate what's happening or berate yourself if you're not relaxing fast enough. We live in such an action-oriented world, this may be difficult when you first start. Just breathe, focus your mind, and let other thoughts come and go as if they are actors walking onstage and you are in the audience, watching. Accept whatever arises—thoughts, feelings, images, and sensations in your body or external noise.

This may not be easy at first, but will become so with time. It's almost as if you step back mentally and allow yourself to be an observer or witness to your thoughts rather than a judge. When you find yourself thinking about everyday thoughts, simply return to your mental or breath focus.

Above all, don't try too hard. Remember that in order to elicit the relaxation response you need to let go. That includes letting go of expectations and goals. Try not to compare one session with another; every relaxation response experience is different. Revel in the variations!

Overcoming Obstacles to Relaxation

Not enough time: If you feel that you are pressed for time and can't possibly fit in twenty minutes in a day, this very lack of time for yourself may be contributing to your symptoms. Remember that you are worth it! Look at your schedule closely. Is there anything that you can drop? You can try two ten-minute sessions sometime during the day. Or try mindfulness. Practice the relaxation response regularly, and you will begin to feel more energized and less frazzled. So just do it! You'll be glad you did.

Can't settle down: If you find that you are jittery and restless, try doing something physical first. Go for a short walk, or take a warm bath or shower. Or try yoga.

You fall asleep: Some people fall asleep while eliciting the relaxation response, especially if they are lying down. This can be a great thing for women suffering from insomnia. Your body is telling you something. Eliciting the relaxation response can be the perfect way to summon sleep. If, however, you are falling asleep before the end of the tape or before fifteen minutes have passed, you will need to add an additional relaxation response practice at another time of day. Sitting upright with your head and neck erect can help you focus and keep you from nodding off.

External distractions: A dog barking, the children fighting, a telephone ringing . . . unless you practice the relaxation response in a soundproof booth, you will hear some external noise during your practice session. Try earplugs or head phones to muffle the sounds. Or visualize the noises as becoming smaller and receding into the horizon. As you exhale, imagine pushing the noises away. Practice noticing them without reacting to them.

Unsettling emotions: Sometimes people find that as they quiet their bodies and try to focus their minds, they become more stressed or anxious. If this happens to you, open your eyes and find a spot or point on which to focus your attention. Take a few deep diaphragmatic breaths. Use visualization if necessary to imagine a warm, safe place. Usually it will pass with time, as you practice the relaxation response more frequently.

If you find very disturbing memories creeping into your consciousness as you practice the relaxation response, or if overwhelming anxiety surfaces and the methods above don't help, you may want to discuss these responses with a health professional or counselor.

"I'm not doing it right": There is no right or wrong way when it comes to the relaxation response. That's why we've suggested a number of techniques and have encouraged you to experiment. If you are able to relax even a little, then you are making progress. Every step toward relaxation is a step in the right direction. Let go of judgments and just notice the experience as it unfolds. As long as you feel better afterwards, you are reaping the benefits.

Body feels different: During a practice session, you may notice that your hands or feet begin to tingle, or that your arms and legs feel heavy. This is actually a sign that you have begun to relax. Try to experience and enjoy the new sensations rather than be distracted by them.

Perhaps the most difficult part of practicing the relaxation response is making it a priority. Many women feel conflicted about making time for such self-nurture. In the next chapter, we'll share some ways to overcome this block and help you make practicing the relaxation response a regular part of your self-care.

CHAPTER 4

Self-Nurture

Have you ever bought a great book only to have it sit on a shelf and gather dust? Or maybe you and a friend have talked about having lunch, only to have conflicting schedules get in the way? The fact is there are many things we plan on doing for ourselves—but never quite get the chance. Throughout this book we discuss a variety of tools and lifestyle approaches for managing your menopause symptoms and improving the quality of your life. But they don't work if you don't use them. For instance, in Chapter 3 we showed you the many ways to elicit the relaxation response. It's proven very effective. But many women come to us and say they can't find the time for it in their busy schedules. Often a lack of time or energy can be a barrier to improving the way we feel. This is where the concept of *self-nurture* comes in.

Self-nurture will help you get the most from this book. It is not a "technique," but rather a mind-set of self-appreciation that frees you to meet your own needs as you continue to care for others. It is not about selfishness or being self-absorbed. On the contrary, it is about fortification. You practice self-nurture by accepting that you deserve the self-care needed to replenish yourself, ignite your spirit, and enliven long-ignored dreams—and by acting on this belief. For example, self-nurture is taking the twenty minutes a day you need to elicit the relaxation response. Women in our programs have found self-nurture sets the stage for a real change in the way they feel and moves them toward discovering and building inner strength.

Self-nurture encompasses nurturing the body, the mind, the emotions, and the spirit. It might include sleeping in, a long walk, enrolling in a yoga class, climbing a mountain, or taking a hot bath by candlelight. There is no one path on the journey of self-nurture. As you read through the book, you'll realize that a daily practice of eliciting the relaxation response, exercise, good nutrition, and the cognitive approaches discussed later in the book (Chapters 10 and 11) are all ways to nurture the self. While the benefits of self-nurture will soon become obvious to you, if you're like many women, you may have trouble actually finding the time for it. The process involves creating time for yourself, setting priorities, learning to listen to what you need, and giving yourself the permission to ask for it. The idea of self-nurture is to find a balance in which you take the deserved time to recharge physically, emotionally, intellectually, creatively, and sensually. It's a journey inward that requires time and space for quiet reflecting. Self-nurture is about hearing your inner voice and listening to what you need. Unfortunately, we cannot begin to count the number of times women in our program have said, "I have no idea what it is that I need." It is in discovering this inner wisdom that women set the stage for feeling better.

Are You a Self-Nurturer?

As each woman is different, so is her approach to life. Some women are inclined to carve out time for themselves, while many others are in desperate need of self-nurture and may not even realize it. Repeatedly women who enter our programs frazzled and fraught with symptoms tell us that once they step back and give themselves permission to nurture themselves they find it much easier to manage many aspects of their lives, including their menopausal symptoms.

For Kara, the stress associated with a high-powered job and juggling many tasks was becoming evident. "I was not taking care of myself. I was putting my husband, my children, my job, and everything else first. My health was suffering. And my quality of life was really in bad shape." Kara, like many of the women in our programs, was experiencing a range of menopausal symptoms; she had trouble sleeping, she was plagued by night sweats, and was worried about her inability to concentrate. These were definitely a source of the problem. But she began to recognize a larger underlying issue: her failure to treat herself in the same way she was culturally taught to care for all of the other significant people in her life. As she began the process of taking time to care for herself, she began to notice a change.

For Helen, the process of self-nurture would begin with a startling revelation. "I didn't think I was worth twenty minutes a day," she flatly recalled. Caught up in the midst of a life filled with a success-oriented husband, a college-aged son, and a highly respected, yet demanding computer programming job, she had been so busy that she did not think about her own needs. What was it that caught her attention? An awareness-building exercise in one of our classes helped bring it to the surface. But it was actually a diagnosis of breast cancer that was the impetus. In seeking out relief from chemotherapy-induced hot flashes, she entered our program hoping to reduce symptoms, but left with an understanding of self-nurture and a new attitude. "It was a life transforming experience. I finally learned I could say no."

Why is it that women often get sick, have trouble coping, or are otherwise at wits' end before they begin to listen to their own needs? Because typically, women will give and give, until they have nothing left to give. Now, consider this. How might *you* benefit from slowing down or reassessing your direction? How many pathways are you taking, and which serve to replenish your soul? This transition can be a time of renewal and regeneration, if you can create the time for self-nurture. The following three-step awareness-buildin¶g exercise is the one we use in our program to help women assess their level of self-nurture. Grab a piece of paper and a pen and try it.

1. Create a "time pie"

If you're one of the many women who lead very busy lives, it may seem that the hours of the day just seem to evaporate. Let's take a look at how you really spend your days. Draw a circle on a sheet of paper. Divide it, pie-like, into segments that represent your average day. Include time for sleep, commuting, work, errands, and other acts that fill your day like watching TV or taking care of pets. Now, label each slice with the activity and number of hours or minutes you spend on it. Be as accurate as possible. If your days are very diverse, create a couple of pies.

Sample Time Pie

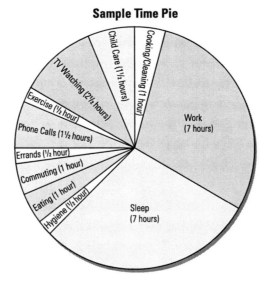

2. Identify what brings you joy

Setting the time pie aside, take a piece of paper and number it from one to twenty. Now, in the next few minutes, quickly jot down twenty things that bring you joy. If you quickly run short of ideas, you're not alone. It is a sad fact that many women actually forget what brings them joy. It has happened many times in our program that we ask women to write down what brings them pleasure or joy. And they can't answer. Deep down they know, but it's been a long time since they've thought about it. If you're having trouble, brainstorm a little. Some of our patients have to reach back to high school or college days to remember what it is that "feeds" their soul. What feeds yours? It doesn't have to be something grand, expensive, or luxurious. It can be as simple as hugging a child or treating yourself to a bouquet of flowers. Try a long soak in the tub with scented candles and bath oils. Maybe you just need a break. Sit in the early morning sun with a book. Stroll along a downtown plaza and window shop. Walk by the water or watch a sunset. Get together with friends and talk about anything but your families and work. Giggle! Go hiking or join a club. Run away to a bed-and-breakfast with your significant other. Think of things that enliven your spirit. Whether conventional or seemingly crazy, add them to your list. If the ideas don't immediately come to you, be open to remembering what brings you joy over the next week. Here are some common joys of women in our programs:

- Time spent with partner
- Music
- A good movie
- Watching a sunset
- The ocean
- Tea in the afternoon (served using the best silver or china)

- Making love
- Girlfriends
- Manicure/pedicure
- Time spent with a pet
- Reading
- Antiquing
- Inline skating
- Streaking my hair
- Buying red high-heeled shoes and a red boa
- Travel
- Finding the nearest national park and exploring
- Walking in a different part of town or in the country each week
- Planting an herb garden or sweet scented flowers indoors or near your back door
- Taking an evening every week to take a class
- Taking your husband out for lunch somewhere new

Next, study your list of all the pastimes and activities that give you pleasure (list of joys) and compare it with your time pie. How many of them appear in both? If you did a chart of a typical week in your life, how many pleasures or joys would appear on that? How about a chart that depicts your typical month? When joys do match up on your "time pie" do they appear in hours or only in minutes? At this point in our awareness-building exercise women often become emotional. They begin to realize that they have neglected certain joys for years, relegating them to the lowest priority. It can be a truly eye-opening exercise—one that may spur you on to make a change.

3. Evaluate the many "slices" of your "pie"

The confusing thing about our schedules is that so much of what we do serves a purpose, especially when it concerns work or family. We are not suggesting you ignore the important things in life. Rather, analyze the many tasks that fill your day. Here's where you can begin to cultivate an attitude of valuing yourself and your needs. Sure there are lots of duties and chores in life. But which tasks, events, or outings really need attending to at the moment, which are truly important, and which ones just seem like it? Often we feel a sense of urgency about some tasks that may not in fact be urgent. The key is knowing the difference.

In his book, *The 7 Habits of Highly Successful People,* Stephen Covey addresses this very issue. He points out that many people routinely choose what seems *urgent* over that which seems *important.* Something that is *important* is valued for itself, philosophically, morally, or ethically. Time spent with a loved one, phoning a friend, practicing the relaxation response, or volunteering may be important to us. But, these activities don't always land on our "to-do" list. They often take a backseat to those things we consider urgent. Generally, we feel something is urgent when there is a real or *imagined* negative outcome if we don't do it. We may believe it's urgent to keep our rooms tidy and our beds made. But when we look back on our lives, will we really yearn for, appreciate, or even remember the times that we made sure we had a spotless house? Or will we wish with regret that we had spent more time with friends, paid more attention to the affections of our child, or did a little more relaxing by the water?

Of course, when there is a true consequence to something urgent (failing to answer the phone when you're expecting news about someone in the hospital, for example), we are not suggesting you ignore that. But when dealing with situations that are perceived as urgent, but are not really—the choice is yours.

Ultimately, we are responsible for our choices. We need to make them thoughtfully. Look at your time pie. How many of the tasks on it are urgent? How many are important? If you feel that you elect to do something because it feels urgent, analyze what would happen if you didn't do it. This can be tremendously helpful, a first step toward freeing up some of your life for *you*.

The Balancing Act

If you find trouble taking time for yourself, you join millions of women who are attempting to do it all. Women today juggle many more roles than ever before in history.

A changing family dynamic is adding to the stress of women, especially at midlife. Women are more frequently in the role of caregiver for aging parents, young or grown children, and grandchildren. Women are typically squeezed between several generations and into multiple roles. It's little wonder that they are increasingly suffering from stress.

As women jump from task to task, the idea of self-nurture may seem like a luxury, even hedonistic. Women often ask us, "When I have so many people around me who need my attention, how can I think of myself?" Added to the stress of juggling roles is often a sense of guilt. One study showed that unlike men, who perceive employment as a normal (and important) part of their role as "parent/breadwinner," many working mothers feel conflicted. They perceive that time at work detracts from their home life and role as nurturing mother or partner. As a result, women feel more guilt about balancing both roles. Stress also appears to affect women differently. A Swedish study, which compared stress levels in men and women, found that women produced higher levels of stress hormones in response to stress and levels of these hormones remained elevated for a longer time.

Alice Domar, Ph.D., a leading expert in stress management for women, spearheaded groundbreaking work on self-nurture while at the Mind/Body Medical Institute. Over her many years working with women, she noticed how a lack of self-nurture affects them. In her book *Self-Nurture,* she comments, "We lack the energy and initiative to solve problems when we're so busy working and taking care of others that we neglect ourselves. We lose commitment to a relaxation practice when we don't feel entitled to even twenty minutes each day for our own well being. We set aside creative pursuits because we internalize negative messages about our talents, or view artistic endeavors as one more drain on our crowded schedule. And, we lose heart when our spiritual growth takes a backseat to duty and obligation. In other words, our inability to self-nurture becomes a roadblock to our efforts to manage stress, enhance health and energy, develop creativity, and cultivate soul."

According to Domar, "Self-nurture is the final pathway, because it grants us the time and space to make the journey inward. With a daily ritual of self-care, an inner worthiness begins to blossom."

Self-Nurture: Getting Started

The concept of self-nurture sounds wonderful in theory. But how do you actually make the time for it and do it? The following steps will help you get started.

Step 1: Define the meaning of self-nurture for *you*

Because self-nurture is a personal journey, there is no one formula. Tailor it to fit your life. If you're balancing a hectic schedule and the idea of self-nurture sounds too time consuming or laughable, try to move away from all-or-nothing thinking. A ten-minute conversation with an old friend can go a long way in making you feel recharged. Self-nurture does not have to take a lot of time or cost any money. The pathways are many. Self-nurture is for women of all walks of life, regardless of ethnicity, income, sexual preference, or background. Inevitably what is joyful for one woman may be drudgery for another. What is possible for one woman may not be possible for another. Several years ago, we had the opportunity to participate in a day-long workshop at an inner city community health center. We were struck by the lives of many of these women. They lived on very little money, cared for families with few resources, and were not in the position to take a getaway. Yet, we found ways they could reap the benefits of self-nurture. During a group brainstorming session, self-nurture was crystallized as spending more time for prayers; setting boundaries that ensure healthy relationships; taking pleasure in a moment of quiet; and maximizing social connections including friends, family, and church.

Here are some ideas generated from women in our groups:

- Notice all your best qualities.
- Have breakfast in bed (preferably served to you) with the Sunday morning paper.
- Rent a movie you've wanted to see.
- Get a massage or facial.
- Buy yourself a bouquet of flowers after a day at work.
- Make time for a hot bath with mineral salts (perhaps by candlelight).
- Allow yourself a good laugh or cry.
- Read the novel that's been sitting by your bed for a year.
- Eat a bowl of ice cream without punishing yourself.
- Leave the dishes; don't make the bed.
- Treat yourself to a haircut and style at a fancy salon.
- Every few months take a mental health day off from your job.
- Say "no" to an invitation you feel obligated to accept on those days when you *really* need a day to yourself.

Create your own list.

Step 2: Change your mind-set

There is irony in the way women approach self-nurture. They highly admire it in other women, but they feel selfish taking time for themselves. Putting the needs of others first is part of the female legacy, handed down from previous generations. Negating thoughts—that it would be selfish, self-centered, self-indulgent, or narcissistic—are common refrains among women who still feel uncomfortable about the idea. We say, "Nonsense! *You are worth it!*"

Cultivating the attitude that you are "worth it" helps free the spirit and lift the guilt. Once you free your thinking about the value of time for you, the next step is to act on your needs.

Step 3: Consider ways to carve out "your" slice of the pie

As you refer back to our time pie exercise, analyze how your own time pie is divided up. If you have noticed that there are no slices left for you, consider making a change. Try reconfiguring your pie to add time for self-nurture. We think it's safe to say that a great book and a hot bubble bath would beat out the eleven o'clock news any day in its ability to de-stress and nourish. Be realistic. And begin to prioritize what's important to you. Here are some ways to accomplish this:

Schedule self-nurture: If you're always on the go, with no time for yourself, you may have to literally schedule time for yourself, date, hour and all. Put it in your planner. When we schedule something, we often feel more committed. If you need encouragement, write down what you need in the form of a prescription. For instance, prescribe a treat like a special cup of tea or coffee or a back rub "to be taken once a day." Prescribe an art class to be taken once a week, or breakfast with a friend every Sunday morning, a half a day without any chores every other weekend, or an hour in the afternoon sitting by the window with a good book.

Divest to invest: In banking, you generally divest from one account or portfolio to invest in another. This is usually done for the good of the individual doing the transaction. Next time you feel the nag by guilt over not doing something for your kids, a friend, or family member, don't think of it as time taken from your loved one. Think of it as adding to a "savings account," which will ultimately benefit them at a later date. When you think of your time to self-nurture as a time to recharge your batteries, it will make sense to you and your family. A large part of this process is *setting boundaries*.

Recall Kara—drained by a busy professional life, lack of sleep, and the needs of her family. As she started working with the group, she learned how to set limits and prioritize. She gave herself permission to spend Sunday mornings in bed (and informed her family of her intention). She would read the paper and sometimes her husband would bring her breakfast in bed. This simple change was one of the most significant and cherished gifts she reaped from the program! And it led to other changes. Sometimes the house cleaning would wait to make room for meditation and relaxation techniques. Kara began to set time aside for exercise, which she thoroughly enjoyed. Her original feelings that she was there to service everyone else began to change. And her family reacted positively when they noticed a change in her mood: "They were really concerned about me. So, when I started taking time for myself and using the relaxation tools, I didn't get a lot of resistance."

In addition, Kara learned how to restructure commitments. One of her daily time stealers and stress producers was her commute to work. When she began to analyze this, she realized that by working a little harder four days of the week, she could work from home on the fifth, allowing her to cut down significantly on commuting time. To get her daughter to soccer matches, she began negotiating carpools (which also helped other mothers).

When you begin to analyze each slice of your daily time pie, certain activities may jump out at you. Others may take some negotiation. By delegating and restructuring duties and obligations, Kara was able to carve more time for herself. She was also less stressed and more present during times with her family. So, think of this the next time that you feel that twinge of guilt. Your family won't notice the tasks you bypass, but will notice when you're fully present in their lives. Today Kara feels more in control. Because she has taken the time to recharge, she has more to give and the time she spends with her family is more fulfilling for everyone.

Work the practice of self-nurture into daily activities: Often women are pleased to find that many of the activities of their typical day are *already* activities that nurture them and bring them joy. Sally discovered that many aspects of her job as a social worker were stimulating and satisfying to her (specifically her interactions with clients) and that others were less fulfilling (paperwork). She noticed she felt better about the day by simply becoming more aware of and present during those enriching parts of her day. Nancy loves nature, so she purposely parks a little further from her office door so that she can take in the flowering trees of spring before sitting down to her computer. Kim, a working single mom, used to feel isolated and alone. Her sister lives only a few blocks away and passes her house twice a day walking her dog. Yet weeks would pass without them seeing each other. Now she meets her sister for fifteen or twenty minutes as often as she can during one of her daily dog-walks. Doing so has allowed her to reduce her feelings of isolation and strengthen her bond with her sister while getting needed exercise. Try adding a self-nurturing twist to each and every day. It helps weave meaning and purpose into our daily lives.

Step 4: Make it "mindful"

Certainly we've eaten a bowl of ice cream and gained nothing more than calories, not even noticing the taste! Self-nurture is not simply engaging in activities we enjoy. Self-nurture is about creating space for and taking pleasure in those things. Thus, there is an element of mindfulness that accompanies a self-nurturing activity. (See Chapter 3 for more on mindfulness.) When we can appreciate the moment of whatever we choose to do, we gain that sense of experience and fulfillment.

A lack of mindfulness is common when we methodically move through our days. For example, it happens when we engage in a conversation, but our thoughts are elsewhere; when we take a shower while making "to do" lists or reliving a fight with our teenager. When we are *not* mindful we lose out on the essence of the experience. When we walk away from a mindful act of self-nurture, whether it's having coffee with an old friend or walking through your backyard, we feel recharged. It is mindfulness that anchors us to the present moment and allows us to fully experience the joy of it.

If, as an adult, you have ever run in the rain, twirled in the sunlight, or gazed at the moon while lying on the grass, you know the powerful impact of a simple act. Yet, for the most part, adults often leave simple acts of joy up to chance or postpone them until "later." As the years pass and obligations build, we fail to pay attention to the multitude of joyful moments in our day and we fail to make time for pleasurable activities. Soon they are slowly crowded out by "to do" lists. As the stress in our life mounts, our desires and creative urges get drowned out by the many voices of duty rushing in. Even planned outings, while enjoyable, can become rife with obligation and duty— especially when laptops and cell phones become part of the luggage.

The power of self-nurture is that meaningful pleasures or moments are not purely left to such a thing as chance. These things become a priority. Time is set aside—sometimes to do nothing—so that when the sun appears, twirling can commence. It's time that does a soul good.

Step 5: Create a "future" time pie

To check your progress and boost your commitment to self-nurture, try creating a "future" time pie that will serve as a goal. Can you add to your list of joys? Have you noticed you have already begun to do so? Some women have commented that just making the list of joys changed their mood. As you begin to reap the benefits of self-nurture, you may be inspired to find a few more "slices" of time.

Step 6: Practice, practice, practice

Remember that it only takes a few moments to de-stress and do something nice for yourself. However, this does not always come naturally, and at first, it takes a commitment. The more you practice incorporating this into your daily life, the more you will realize that self-nurture can truly pave the way for a renaissance of the spirit and a strengthening of the soul. It can lead you to quiet and calm and help you to best figure out how to listen to what it is you need to enrich your life and feel better.

Self-Nurture and Relationships

You may be wondering: how can I focus on myself without alienating the people in my life? Nurturing ourselves in the context of our relationships is a part of self-nurture. This involves defining time for ourselves and stating what we need from others. Once we begin to ponder our needs, we can begin to meet them in a healthy way. If you need more recognition for your work (on the job or at home), let those who can best give you positive feedback know that you need it. If you think your sexual needs are not being met, express what you need to your partner.

Sometimes those closest to us may not be aware of our limits or needs. If we do not express our needs, it can often lead to misunderstanding, resentment, and even anger. On the other hand, when we learn to communicate our needs and limits, it can create a balance that can ultimately make both parties happier. Try aspiring for the best of both—quality time with yourself and others.

When you're planning your calendar, are you planning social events (dinners, etc.) out of obligation or desire? Knowing the difference may help you make self-nurturing decisions. If you can, ease out of events that leave you feeling drained. Use the time you save to carve out a meaningful intimate dinner with an old friend. Treat your daily interactions with loved ones with the same exuberance. Instead of thinking of mealtime with your family as a chore, use it as a time to truly explore the feelings of the other family members. Enjoy the taste of the food, gaze into the eyes of your husband, kids, or significant other, and tell them something great.

"Acts of kindness": Want to enjoy an easy way of getting your needs met while strengthening bonds with your significant other? Try an exercise that can provide you both with strength and compassion when you need it most. This simple but effective idea came from one of our patients. Create a list of twenty acts of kindness you would appreciate from your partner. Have your partner do the same. Then, when either you or your partner has had a particularly emotional, stressful, or exhausting day, ask for one of the acts of kindness from your lists. It's a great exercise because it tells your partner when you're stressed or exhausted and you get your partner's support when you need it most, which will ultimately improve your relationship. You might want to include the following examples of "acts of kindness" from Alice Domar's book *Self-Nurture*:

- Prepare dinner and clean up with no help from me whatsoever.

- Read aloud to me from an inspirational book on spiritual coping.
- Pick up a video rental of a romantic movie and watch it with me.
- Buy me a bouquet of fresh-cut flowers.
- Buy a box of expensive chocolates and have it ready.
- Pick up a bowl of chicken soup and bring it to me in bed, even though I'm not sick.
- Insist that I stay off my feet and relax, and do anything and everything to make certain I stay that way for the rest of the day/evening.
- Sit and listen to me complain without saying one word for twenty minutes.
- Call back my mother/father/sister/brother and tell them I can't come to the phone right now because I am too exhausted.
- Pour me a glass of chilled wine and bring it here pronto.
- Take care of the children without any help whatsoever from me.
- Let me literally cry on your shoulder.
- Go out and buy me the pair of shoes I've been staring at in the store window for weeks.
- Pull me out of my misery by taking me for a walk or drive to my favorite park or nature preserve.
- Allow us to spend the next hour together in blissful silence.
- Massage my feet while I watch the film of my choice on TV.
- Take me to my favorite restaurant and act as if we were on an early romantic date.
- Plant kisses on the back of my neck.
- Tell me why you were so attracted to me when we first met.

"Good for you" getaways: One of Sheila's self-nurturing acts has been to schedule regular vacations with her husband, leaving the kids at home. "I come back and I'm completely de-stressed!" Getaways with no agendas or obligations can be highly rewarding. Think of all the ways you can nurture yourselves as a couple and as individuals. In addition to scheduling getaways with her husband, Sheila got season tickets to the ballet, a rare treat. As she sees it, "It's a way of eliciting the relaxation response. I am mindful and feel like I am at complete peace."

Nurturing Your Many "Selves"

We can find our own style of being, relating, and creating that makes us glad to get up in the morning, one that feeds our zest and enthusiasm for life. Nurturing our creative selves means opening our minds and hearts to the sea of possibilities, to heed the inner voice of imagination.

—LAWRENCE LESHAN

Once you have begun to make self-nurture a part of your life, you will start to realize that there are many ways to nurture yourself and that they involve different aspects of your life. Nurturing the many aspects of our "selves" promotes health; it creates balance in our lives. In a sense, we diversify our lives and ourselves in a good way—one that builds self-esteem and ultimately buffers stress and illness as well. When we cultivate our "multiple selves" (mother, career woman, friend, partner, artist) we become more resilient to stress. Thus, the woman who has strong friendships, is part of a choir, and is involved in meaningful community action projects, for example, will not be as rattled if there is a crisis in one part of her life (for example, at work) as the woman whose whole life is defined by work. When the chips are down in one facet of our lives, we are sustained by the sources of pride, joy, or accomplishment in other parts of our lives.

Often various ways of self-nurturing lead to a process of self-discovery and combine to allow for a new outlook on life. Helen, who felt her life was being disrupted by hot flashes, began a serious yoga practice and started eliciting the relaxation response daily. Eventually feelings of resentment made way for feelings of control. Helen began to notice a change: "I still have hot flashes, but they don't bother me as much anymore." Taking the time to self-nurture has also allowed her to tap into her talents, find new ways of expression, and bond with friends. She now regularly meets with friends for coffee just to talk, and she has begun watercolor painting classes, something she has always wanted to do. "I love it. I have begun to take over my post-child life for myself. What's different about me is all nonverbal. The fundamentally transforming thing is discovering that I'm worth that time."

How do we best realize our strengths? Nurturing your many "selves" is about learning to care for yourself in a way that will lead to a deep appreciation and commitment to all aspects of self: mind, body, emotions, and spirit. When you set a regular RR practice as a priority, when you commit yourself to becoming a more active person, when you find a balance for healthful eating, the journey toward postmenopausal health and quality of life is yours.

We end this chapter with one of the most basic and for many women neglected aspects of self-nurture—the spiritual self. What is it that feeds your soul? This encompasses creative endeavors as well as the more fundamental concept: our deepest self. The wisdom of the ancients tells us: "our deepest self is our highest self." How can you use self-nurture to help you reach and replenish your inner wisdom? Start by unleashing your spiritual and creative "selves."

Nurturing your creativity: It seems the vibrant beauty of color, the magic of acting, the sound of music, and words from the heart all have the power to transform us. If you have spent your life dedicated to family, work, and friends, chances are you have not fully explored your inner well of creativity. You may not even know your true potential. For this reason, your forties, fifties, and beyond can be a time of profound growth and freedom. It has been said that postmenopausal zest often heralds a surging of emotion and creativity. You have likely always had inner talents, just not taken the time or space to fully explore them! Self-nurture can be the vehicle to open the imagination to life and plant seeds of creativity. To begin to nurture your creative self, try taking a class. Whether it's pottery, drawing, or any type of hobby, it's a great way to get started. If you don't have time for class, pick up a few supplies at an art store and dabble whenever you have a few moments. Buy yourself a new journal and spend some time every day writing. Treat yourself to piano lessons. Or think about

Ignite Your Artistic Spark

Like our cars, lost hidden talents may need the proverbial "jump-start." Julia Cameron, author of *The Artist's Way,* has an exercise called "buried dreams" that may prompt you in realizing your inner artist. As she points out, it may take some excavating:

Buried Dreams
Note: when doing this exercise be fast and frivolous. This is an exercise in spontaneity, so be sure to write your answers out quickly. As she points out, speed kills the censor.

1. List five hobbies that sound fun.
2. List five classes that sound fun.
3. List five things you personally would *never* do that sound fun.
4. List five skills that would be fun to have.
5. List five things you used to enjoy doing.
6. List five silly things you would like to try once.

Try acting on buried dreams. You never know.

treating yourself as often as you can to a visit to a museum or take in a community play.

Nurture your spirituality: There is no one path to spirituality. For many of us, this is not necessarily a religious path. It is a path of "connection." We can offer guidance, but ultimately the journey of discovering and embracing the spiritual self is a personal one. There are lots of meanings to spirituality. We believe that each woman can find a sense of spirituality that is meaningful to her, and that this ultimately can improve her health and well-being.

Over the years, in our programs ranging from cardiac, to cancer, to HIV, to chronic pain, to infertility and menopause, we have worked with thousands of patients with many different personal belief systems. For some of these patients spirituality is related to a formal religion, for some it is nature. As varied as are our many patients, so is the concept of spirituality.

In our programs, we use the following definition:

Spirituality: The belief that on a profound level one feels connected to oneself and to others. The belief that one's life has meaning and purpose.

The journey is to find that connection for yourself. For some it comes with belonging to church or synagogue, for some it is watching a sunset, or being on a mountaintop. For others it is found in meditation and journeying inward to develop a deep connection to self. And for some it may be the smile on your child's face, or the work you do for others.

An inner retreat: There is an ancient way of attaining knowledge that bolsters spirituality and puts one in touch with the inner world. Called a *vision quest,* it has been used by Native Americans to gain spiritual guidance and inner strength. Today vision quests have become popular forms of retreat. Typically, they involve a journey into the wilderness and days of personal and spiritual reflection. While we can't offer advice on trekking off into the great outdoors, we can encourage you to take what Dr. Domar calls a "personal retreat," one that is simple and self-nurturing. What's great is that you don't have to go far to journey inward! The directions are simply stated in an ancient teaching:

Learn to be silent. Let your quiet mind listen and absorb.

—PYTHAGORAS

If you can, clear a weekend or even a few hours, and use the time for inner care: meditation, contemplation, relaxation, and mindful acts of enjoying nature. Whether you choose to take a trip to a natural area or simply stay at home, doesn't matter. Wherever you are, set the stage for relaxation and inspiration. If at home take long naps, hot baths, and try aromatherapy. Clear your mind, cut out television, magazines, newspapers, and any reading material that is not spiritually rewarding. Even a few hours of undivided self-nurture can be greatly rejuvenating. If you can get the house to yourself, even better. Solitude is great for clearing the mind.

If you choose to use nature as your backdrop, simply look around! While struggling with the mood swings of perimenopause, Holly began to take outings into her own backyard. "It changed how I felt psychologically. I learned to appreciate more. Today, I appreciate and enjoy a beautiful spring day simply because it's beautiful." The time in her own backyard has allowed Holly a certain silence, a chance to look inward for strength and outward for beauty.

Making choices: Living the life you want

As you go forward, read this book with the idea of self-nurture in mind. Nurturing the mind, body, and spirit can be an experience of profound growth and liberation. It can open new doorways and pro-

Wise Person Guided Imagery

Wouldn't it be nice to have a sage to present all your problems to? Using this guided imagery exercise you can increase your awareness of inner wisdom and connection to "self." Think of a pressing problem. Begin to elicit the relaxation response with a breath focus or body scan (see Chapter 3) and once your mind is quiet consider the following imagery.

Imagine walking along a mountain path on a journey you have long awaited, for at the end of this path is a wise and compassionate person. You have heard of this person's keen insights and loving nature and have hoped that one day you would meet. Today is the day. Over the next few minutes allow yourself to experience the splendor of anticipation as you climb in mindfulness focusing your attention on your sensory experience. Within your imagination, it is likely your favorite season and your favorite time of day. As you progress, gently notice the sights around you.

> Breathe in the fragrances.
> Notice the tastes unique to this place.
> And now allow yourself to focus on the sounds.

Now gently bring your awareness on your sense of touch. Perhaps you've found a mountain stream for your refreshment. Over the next few moments continue along your path, letting your attention dwell in this way on any or all of your senses.

In a few moments your path will end and you will see a cottage or dwelling of some kind with a welcome sign. Upon entering the dwelling you are greeted by this most wise and compassionate person. Allow yourself to become familiar with him/her in any way that feels comfortable. Then begin to describe your concern or problem. Sit in the silence. Listen to this wise person's guidance and engage in a dialogue to aid your understanding.

In the next few moments say goodbye in any way that feels right. You may choose to make another appointment to meet in the near future. And when you feel ready, begin your journey back down the mountain reflecting upon the significance of your experience.

mote a "zestful" life in the years to come. As Kara has found, embracing self-nurture involves some degree of letting go. "I don't feel like I have to have a perfectly clean, organized house. I try to savor the time I have at home. If I have the choice between running an errand and going on a beach walk, I go on a beach walk." Kara has enhanced her life by working to achieve a balance between career, family, and self. Like many of us, she is managing to match a tendency to do a lot with a prescription for inner calm. "I have learned to do nothing."

Indeed, in clearing our schedules and leaving our closets messy, we may just allow time for the life we want.

CHAPTER 5

Exercise:
Moving Through Menopause

If a friend approached you claiming she was able to control her weight, improve sleep, boost her mood, sharpen her mental functioning, and improve her sex life, chances are you'd want to follow her every move. Robert Butler, M.D., of the International Longevity Center sums it up nicely: "If exercise could be put in a pill, it would be the most widely prescribed medicine in the world."

Women consistently say exercise has a profound effect on the way they feel during and after the menopause transition. Despite this, getting motivated to exercise is sometimes a hurdle, especially for women with busy schedules. The U.S. surgeon general recommends that people do moderate exercise at least thirty (preferably sixty if weight loss is an issue) minutes a day, most days a week. It can be as simple as yard work or playing with the dog. Yet fewer than one in three Americans meets the minimum recommendations and another four in ten American adults participate in no physical activity during their leisure time, even though decades of research confirm that exercise improves health and can extend your life. In this chapter, we'll explain how regular exercise can help you move through menopause with more ease and comfort. What's more, we hope to convince you that exercise is a gift, not a burden. We want it to become something you *want* to do, rather than something you *have* to do. It will become a treasured time-out from the demands of the day, one that you can't imagine doing without. For Michelle, exercise, specifically running, has been a way of life. "There is a runner's high that you get," she says. She thinks of time on the open road as a getaway of sorts. "It's the repetition in running that helps you zone out." Michelle maintains a regular workout routine, incorporating strength training and aerobics. What keeps her going is that it makes her feel so good. As she begins to move, she goes through a transformation: "I feel my shoulders loosen up and my whole body feels better."

A Mind/Body Perspective on Exercise

If you exercise only to lose weight, you're missing part of a much larger picture. Exercise also has a powerful effect on the mind. It triggers the release of powerful endorphins, which have been described as prompting feelings of elation or calm.

Exercise also helps you get in touch with your innermost self: your spirit or soul. This is especially true when it is combined with the relaxation response (RR) we explored in detail in Chapter 3. When exercise is used to elicit the RR, the result is a tremendous release of tension and an enhanced feeling of well-being.

The key to developing this approach to exercise is to shift your focus away from specific goals (number of calories burned or minutes spent exercising) and instead focus on the process: how you feel as you move. To help maintain this state of mind use the two components central to eliciting the RR—a repetitive focus (breath, a mantra, or a physical rhythm) and a nonjudging attitude (accepting the experience as it happens) when you exercise.

To exercise your spirit by eliciting the RR, any physical activity will do as long as it has the following characteristics:

- It's enjoyable
- It's noncompetitive or nonjudgmental
- It's predictable and provides a sense of safety and reliability
- It's repetitive and rhythmic so you can focus your awareness
- It involves abdominal breathing, the key to relaxation
- It lasts for twenty to thirty minutes

Many exercises embody these characteristics, including yoga, swimming, and walking. Aerobic exercise particularly helps elicit the RR because it involves deep breathing and a particular rhythm. Whatever activity you choose, remember to adopt a nonjudging attitude and an inward focus as you do it.

How does this attitude shift take place? One important step is to learn to regard physical activity as a way of reinvigorating your mind as well as your body. Our mind/body program for menopause offers a holistic approach to exercise that is based on the premise that mind and body are not separate; instead, they are different expressions of the fundamental life force.

Our holistic approach involves three key elements. Two elements—cardiovascular activities for endurance and musculoskeletal exercises for strength and flexibility—will sound familiar. It's the third element—body awareness—that makes our program unique. Body awareness involves paying attention to what you are feeling while you exercise. If you learn to listen to your body, and respond to how you feel, you will know when to ease off and take it easy, and when to push a little harder. You will learn to listen to the messages you receive from your body as you move, and to make choices based on what you hear.

This approach to exercise not only tones your body, it facilitates

The Elements of Holistic Exercise

A mind/body approach to exercise encompasses the traditional elements of exercise, but also adds an additional element: body awareness. This approach requires adopting a different mind-set toward exercise than you may be used to. For one thing, the focus is on listening to the messages from your body rather than trying to meet an external goal (such as number of minutes or calories burned). Decisions about how long or how hard to exercise are based on feedback from your body. This facilitates self-knowledge and acceptance, relieves stress, and reduces risk of injury.

Type of Exercise	Traditional View	Holistic Mind/Body View
AEROBIC EXERCISE (Examples: walking, swimming, bicycling)	• Builds cardiovascular fitness • Increases endurance • Enables you to be physically active for extended periods without experiencing fatigue	• Keep focus internal • Focus on breath rhythm and deep abdominal breathing • Focus on cadence of steps while walking or jogging, on pedaling while riding a bicycle, or on arm strokes while swimming

self-acceptance and self-knowledge. As physician and runner George Sheehan wrote, "The body mirrors the mind and soul and is much more accessible than either. If you can become proficient at listening to your body, you will eventually hear from your whole self."

Following this approach, exercise becomes a means of self-observation and a way to increase self-awareness rather than just something you have to suffer through to meet a goal. When you begin to view exercise as a way of life, and not as an obligation, then you are truly on the path to improving your physical and spiritual health.

Type of Exercise	Traditional View	Holistic Mind/Body View
MUSCULOSKELETAL EXERCISES (Examples: lifting weights, muscle stretches)	• Increases muscle strength • Increases overall flexibility • Reduces risk of injury during normal daily tasks	• Movements are slow and rhythmic, coordinated with breathing • Focus is internal on how the muscles feel as they move • Uses yoga to realign posture, release tension, and maintain a basic "resting state" • Uses tai chi as a "moving meditation," to provide focus for the body and mind

Exercise to Improve Menopausal Symptoms

In the fifth century BC, Hippocrates wrote, "Eating alone will not keep a man well; he must also take exercise. For food and exercise, while possessing opposite qualities, yet work together to produce health." For women, exercise can be a soothing balm in the face of tension, an invigorating release in the presence of hormonal disruptions, and a way to preserve the physical freedoms we all associate with youth. Exercise holds so many benefits for the menopausal woman that we consider it an essential part of our program.

What's more, exercise mimics a "fountain of youth" in a number of ways. Studies have shown that much of the physical deterioration that takes place between ages thirty and seventy is related to a sedentary lifestyle, not the aging process. Exercising does its magic by slowing deterioration of various body systems. It can help reverse problems associated with the so-called "normal" aging process, such as loss of muscle strength and bone mass, and impairments in sleep, sex, and cognitive function. Even many of the physical changes generally associated with menopause may actually be a product of inactivity and not solely hormones.

Many women report that exercise improves PMS symptoms and hot flashes while boosting body image and mood. It's also great for maintaining bone density and helps maintain balance and flexibility, which decreases your risk for falls and fractures as you get older.

Hot flashes: Many women report that regular workouts help reduce the number of hot flashes and night sweats. And there are data to support their observations. In 1990, a Swedish study followed 142 women going through natural menopause, without hormone therapy. Women known to exercise regularly reported half the number of moderate and severe hot flashes as did women who did not exercise regularly. Eight years later, research from University Hospital, Linköping, added to the data. In this research, only 5 percent of very active women experienced severe hot flashes as compared with 14–16 percent of women who were sedentary. Weight, smoking, or hormone therapy couldn't explain the difference. Certainly it's possible that there's something about women who exercise regularly that makes them less prone to (or less bothered by) hot flashes. However, there is also a potential physical explanation: regular exercise affects the brain chemicals responsible for regulating body temperature.

Exercise offers a natural way to fend off hot flashes, with lots of extra benefits and virtually no downside.

PMS symptoms: A small study from Duke University examined the effects of aerobic exercise and strength training in healthy premenopausal women. After three months, the women who exercised not only experienced fitness gains, but they also had less severe PMS symptoms. And aerobic exercise appeared more beneficial than strength training, particularly for PMS-related depression. In another study, one group of women participated in a running program—half of them had not exercised regularly before the study; the other half were regular exercisers and ramped up their running to train for a marathon. The second group of women was normally active, but did not undertake an aerobic training program of any kind. After six months, all of the exercisers reported less fluid retention, depression, and anxiety than did the nonexercisers.

These were small studies, but many women report that regular aerobic exercise helps them manage PMS. How might exercise make a difference? First, it boosts endorphins. These neurotransmitters can improve mood and sense of well-being. Other possible benefits include stable blood sugar levels, which might help reduce cravings, improve energy, and reduce stress and anxiety.

Mood swings: For many women, exercise can put the brakes on a bad mood, anger, depression, and anxiety. "I know I feel better when I exercise. If time goes by and I can't, I can feel the tension in my body. The tension makes the stress worse and stress makes the hormones worse," said one woman in our program.

This reaction to exercise underscores the important mind/body connection mentioned above. Aerobic exercise prompts the release of mood-lifting hormones and neurotransmitters, which relieve stress and promote a sense of well being. Duke University scientists even found that regular aerobic exercise could be as effective as an antidepressant drug in reducing symptoms of depression in older individuals. A follow-up study found that people who continued to exercise not only continued to benefit, but were also less likely than those on medication to suffer a relapse of depressive symptoms.

Because of our cultural obsession with young and beautiful bodies, some women fear that menopause signals a loss of attractiveness and vitality. For women at midlife, regular exercise has been shown to improve body satisfaction, self-confidence, and sense of control, and decrease anxiety associated with body image.

Improved sleep: Exercise facilitates sleep by producing a significant rise in body temperature, followed by a compensatory drop a few hours later. The drop in body temperature, which persists for two to four hours after exercise, makes it easier to fall asleep and stay asleep. An extra benefit of quality sleep: improved mood.

Controlling weight changes: As they age, many women also find they put on pounds where they never had before, especially in the stomach and waist. Exactly what causes this is unclear. The end of ovarian function may influence how the body stores fat. Unfortunately, this switch to abdominal fat storage is associated with increased heart disease and may be one reason a postmenopausal woman's risk of heart disease increases to match that of a man. People who are "apple shaped," that is they put on extra fat around the middle, are more likely to experience certain health problems compared to people who are "pear shaped" and carry extra weight in their hips and thighs.

Women at any age are generally at a disadvantage compared to men when it comes to keeping the pounds off. The following physiological differences between men and women help explain why women do have to work a little harder.

- Women tend to store fat in their hips, thighs, and buttocks. This is the hardest type of fat to lose, since fat metabolism in this part of the body is less robust than in the upper abdominal region, where men tend to store fat. Women can lose fat, but it generally takes more effort.
- Women tend to have a resting metabolic rate that is 5–10 percent lower than that of men's. Because of the lower metabolic rate, women tend to burn calories more slowly.
- The average American woman has 36 percent body fat, while

the typical man has 23 percent. (The amount considered normal is about half that amount: 18–22 percent for women, and 12–15 percent for men.) Because muscle burns more calories than fat, this type of body composition also slows weight loss in women.

- Due to their lower resting metabolism and higher percentage of body fat, when women exercise, they burn up to 40 percent fewer calories than men doing the same activity.

Many women complain they have a harder time controlling weight as they get older. In general, women tend to add more body fat and lose more muscle than men do over the years. Research shows this is because women, in general, become less active as they age. Increasing exercise would help women close this gap.

Regular physical activity, done over a prolonged period, will reshape your body by building muscle, boosting your metabolism, and burning fat. The more muscle you have, the more calories you burn all day long, so lowering your percentage of body fat while increasing muscle is an investment that pays off throughout the day.

Prescription for Weight Loss

To maximize your chances of losing weight, aim for the following:

- Exercise for forty to sixty minutes per day (enough to burn three hundred to four hundred calories a session).
- Choose moderate-intensity activities.
- Exercise four to seven times a week (the higher the frequency, the more important it is to do cross-training to decrease your risk of injury).
- Pick activities that involve large muscle groups, such as the legs, rather than smaller muscles such as the arms.
- Include weight training as well as aerobic activities.

The "Anti-Aging" Benefits of Exercise

If you want to feel young, rest is not the prescription. Here are the determinants of aging that you can control:

- *Muscle mass:* The rate at which you lose muscle mass accelerates after age forty-five. Use your muscles frequently and they'll stay stronger, rather than shrinking.
- *Strength:* After age thirty—perhaps as early as age twenty—you lose both muscle cells and the nerve connections that tell them to contract. To preserve these, apply the "use it or lose it" rule.
- *Basal metabolic rate (BMR):* The number of calories you burn at rest, known as your basal metabolic rate, drops starting at age twenty. Generally, that's because older people have less fat-free mass (muscle and bone), a major contributor to BMR. Build muscle and bone and you burn more calories.
- *Body fat percentage:* The average twenty-five-year-old woman is 25 percent fat. The average sixty-five-year-old woman is 43 percent fat. Cutting calories can help you lose fat, but unless you exercise you'll also lose muscle. Maintaining muscle will help prevent you from gaining fat.
- *Aerobic capacity:* The better your ability to perform a moderate, sustained activity (such as walking, running, or cycling), the lower your risk of heart disease, diabetes, and even colon cancer.
- *Blood-sugar tolerance:* When it's low, you have a higher risk of heart disease

The Long-Term Health Benefits of Exercise

A sedentary lifestyle can be deadly. More than one in ten deaths in this country—250,000 per year—are caused by lack of regular physical activity.

Whether you are worried about cancer, heart attacks, or the life-altering impacts of osteoporosis, you will find few better preventive treatments than adopting a healthy lifestyle that includes exercise.

and diabetes. Maintain your tolerance with a low-fat, high-fiber diet and exercise, which lowers body fat and helps prevent large swings in blood sugar and insulin levels.

- *Cholesterol and triglyceride levels:* Exercise can help improve your cholesterol profile by raising levels of HDL ("good" cholesterol) and lowering levels of triglycerides, which can increase your risk for heart disease.

- *Blood pressure:* Some studies show that people who exercise have a lower risk of high blood pressure, and exercise has been found to help lower blood pressure in people who have high blood pressure.

- *Bone density:* Weight-bearing exercise (strength training, running, and walking) can reduce the rate at which you lose bone. As our muscles pull on our bones and our bones lift our body weight or support weight-bearing activities, the bones are stressed. To adapt, they grow stronger.

- *Body-temperature regulation:* Older people are more susceptible to dehydration and injuries caused by heat or cold. Regular exercise increases blood volume, which increases circulating fluids and helps prevent dehydration. (It's still important to drink plenty of fluids!) Aerobic exercise also makes you sweat, which serves to cool the body down.

Source: Adapted from ten "biomarkers" list created by William Evans, Ph.D. (USDA's Human Nutrition Research Center on Aging at Tufts University) and Irwin Rosenberg, M.D.

Heart disease: The more physically fit you are, the lower your chances of developing heart disease or suffering a heart attack. In fact, a recent study found that low exercise capacity may be as powerful a predictor of mortality as other cardiac risk factors such as high blood pressure, smoking, and diabetes.

Diabetes: Exercise can help to prevent the development of non-insulin-dependent diabetes and the accompanying risk to your heart. Exer-

Accurate Measurements

You can't rely on the scale to tell you if an exercise program is working because weighing yourself doesn't measure body composition or body fat. You can actually lose inches around your waist and put on weight because muscle is more dense than fat (a pound of muscle takes up less space than a pound of fat).

Instead of counting pounds, keep track of your waist size over the years. To do this, stand up straight, hold one end of a tape measure at about the navel, and measure all the way around the waist. Taking this measurement regularly will help you accurately chart positive and negative changes.

Another way to judge if you're a healthy weight is to measure your body mass index (BMI). This calculation takes into account height and weight (see chart). Women with a BMI of 30 or higher or who have a waist size of 35 inches or larger are at particularly high risk for health problems related to obesity, including heart disease and diabetes.

cise appears to make cells more sensitive to insulin, the hormone that regulates the uptake of glucose into the cells.

"Syndrome X": Hormonal changes at menopause increase a woman's risk of developing several of the conditions that help define "Syndrome X" (insulin resistance, high blood pressure, high triglycerides, decreased HDL, and abdominal obesity). Syndrome X increases your risk for diabetes and heart disease. People with three or more of the following are considered to have Syndrome X: abdominal obesity (waist circumference larger than 35 inches in women); triglycerides higher than or equal to 150 mg/dL; HDL cholesterol lower than 50 mg/dL; blood pressure over 130/85 mmHg, and fasting glucose over 110 mg/dL. Diet and exercise have been found to improve the metabolic condition.

Blood clots: Regular exercise reduces the risk that you will develop a blood clot. It appears that regular physical activity enhances the ef-

Determining Your Body Mass Index

	WEIGHT															
HEIGHT	100	110	120	130	140	150	160	170	180	190	200	210	220	230	240	250
5'0"	20	21	23	25	27	29	31	33	35	37	39	41	43	45	47	49
5'1"	19	21	23	25	26	28	30	32	34	36	38	40	42	43	45	47
5'2"	18	20	22	24	26	27	29	31	33	35	37	38	40	42	44	46
5'3"	18	19	21	23	25	27	28	30	32	34	35	37	39	41	43	44
5'4"	17	19	21	22	24	26	27	29	31	33	34	36	38	39	41	43
5'5"	17	18	20	22	23	25	27	28	30	32	33	35	37	38	40	42
5'6"	16	18	19	21	23	24	26	27	29	31	32	34	36	37	39	40
5'7"	16	17	19	20	22	23	25	27	28	30	31	33	34	36	38	39
5'8"	15	17	18	20	21	23	24	26	27	29	30	32	33	35	36	38
5'9"	15	16	18	19	21	22	24	25	27	28	30	31	32	34	35	37
5'10"	14	16	17	19	20	22	23	24	26	27	29	30	32	33	34	36
5'11"	14	15	17	18	20	21	22	24	25	26	27	28	30	32	33	35
6'0"	14	15	16	18	19	20	22	23	24	26	27	28	30	31	33	34
6'1"	13	15	16	17	18	20	21	22	24	25	26	28	29	30	32	33
6'2"	13	14	15	17	18	19	21	22	23	24	26	27	28	30	31	32
6'3"	12	14	15	16	17	19	20	21	22	24	25	26	27	29	30	31
6'4"	12	13	15	16	17	18	19	21	22	23	24	26	27	28	29	30

To estimate your body mass index (BMI), first identify your weight (to the nearest 10 pounds) in the top row of the chart. Next, move your finger down the column below that weight until you come to the row that represents your height. The number at the intersection of your height and weight is your BMI.

BMI	Interpretation
Under 18.5	Underweight
18.5–24	Normal
25–29	Overweight
30 and above	Obese

fects of natural anticlotting chemicals in the blood and prevents blood platelets from sticking together.

Cancer: Several lines of evidence support regular low-to-moderate-intensity physical activity as a preventive strategy for certain cancers. Of particular interest to menopausal women are data from the Nurses' Health Study, a large observational study that has shown that postmenopausal women who engaged in at least one hour of physical activity a day were 15–20 percent less likely to develop breast cancer than women who didn't exercise. Indeed, of all lifestyle factors, a lack of physical activity is the one most consistently linked to a heightened risk for colorectal cancer. A 1997 study, involving both men and women, showed that people who exercised vigorously during at least three different periods of their lives had a 40 percent lower risk of developing the disease. Data from the Nurses' Health Study, also published in 1997, made the equation even more specific: middle-aged American women who participated in approximately four hours of moderate or three hours of intense activity each week cut their chances of developing colon cancer in half. Nurses' Health Study researchers also estimate that more than 15 percent of all colorectal cancers could be prevented if people added half an hour of walking to their daily routine.

Osteoporosis and falls: Physical activity places mechanical stress on your bones, which helps build new, stronger bone. What's more, regular exercise increases muscle strength, balance, and flexibility, all of which prevents falls (and thus fractures).

Cognitive functions: Exercise improves the heart's ability to pump blood more effectively, and increases the blood's oxygen-carrying ability. Because of this, some people believe that exercise might be able to offset some of the mental declines that we often associate with aging by increasing blood flow and oxygen to the brain. A study from the University of Illinois studied 124 adults between the ages of sixty and seventy-five. Half were assigned to a walking program, the other to a stretching program. After six months, not only did the walkers have better cardiovascular fitness, but they also did better on cognitive tests. Duke University researchers confirmed these findings in a study that showed exercise improves "executive functions" such as planning and organizing skills.

Boosting immunity: Although we don't know all the ways that exercise affects immune system function, it's clear that people who exercise regularly don't become ill as often as sedentary people. It appears that moderate physical activity triggers the release of hormones that stimulate the immune system, which, in turn, increases the numbers and activities of certain protective cells. Some of these protective cells include natural killer cells that are part of the body's defense against viruses and malignancies. This may help explain why regular exercise reduces the risk of certain cancers. However, these benefits appear to be lost when people exercise at high intensity, such as training for or running a marathon.

An Exercise Plan: Getting Started

So how much exercise do you need, and what kind should you do, in order to reap all these wonderful benefits? The federal government has established minimum guidelines on physical activity based on a number of studies that we'll discuss in the pages that follow. These recommendations may seem at first to contradict our earlier advice of letting go of goals. Our philosophy, however, is quite simple: know what you're aiming for, but go with the flow of what feels right for you and remember that *something is better than nothing*. All too often, people who have led mainly sedentary lives are intimidated by the thought of suddenly committing themselves to an exercise regimen. So whatever you do, start slowly and build gradually over a matter of weeks or even months if that is what it takes.

Building a fitness foundation

In the 1970s and 1980s, many health care professionals believed the common refrain "no pain, no gain." The recommendations for exercise were so demanding that many Americans just couldn't meet them,

Medical Considerations

Health problems are not reasons to exclude exercise from your lifestyle. In fact, as we have already mentioned, the opposite is true. However, you may need to modify exercises to prevent stress and injury. If you have heart disease, osteoporosis, a pulmonary or metabolic disease, or two or more of the risk factors listed below, consult your doctor before starting a new exercise program:

- High blood pressure
- Elevated cholesterol
- Cigarette smoking
- Abnormal resting EKG
- Family history of heart disease before age fifty
- Diabetes
- Thyroid disorders
- Kidney disease
- Liver disease
- Older than fifty

got discouraged, and gave up. However, scientists from the Centers for Disease Control and Prevention and the American College of Sports Medicine convened a panel in the mid-1990s to review the evidence on exercise. They concluded that moderate exercise offered people the most overall health benefits, and that the number of calories expended on exercise per week mattered more than the intensity, length, or type of activity. As a result, the scientists issued a new set of guidelines that can be summarized by "less pain, more gain."

Follow these recommendations, and you will be well on your way to building a foundation for fitness:

- Accumulate thirty minutes or more of moderate-intensity physical activity on most (or all) days of the week; aim for three to four hours a week. If weight loss is a goal, you may need to do closer to sixty minutes.

- Ten-minute bouts of activity done three times a day are just as good as a continuous half-hour activity. For example, you could do a brisk fifteen-minute walk before going to work, then park your car ten minutes away from your office and walk that distance briskly in the morning. Then walk briskly back to your car at the end of the day. That's thirty-five minutes of activity. Be flexible so you can make adjustments as needed. If it's going to rain two days in a row, think of an indoor location where you can walk during lunch or at the end of the day. Or plan to walk for longer periods once the sun comes back out so that you still achieve your weekly goal.

- Aim to burn 1,000 to 1,400 calories a week during exercise, the number of calories expended per week found to correlate with health benefits. Walking briskly for thirty minutes (or an equivalent level of exercise) will expend 150–200 calories.

- Any activity is good if it gets you moving. But if you're doing a low-intensity activity, do it for a longer period of time than you would a high-intensity exercise so you burn enough calories.

All sorts of activities count as you build your foundation of fitness: formal activities like aerobics or weight lifting at a gym; informal activities like walking up the stairs instead of taking the elevator;

Whether you're a beginner or a seasoned fitness expert, walking is an ideal aerobic activity for most people. It doesn't require any special equipment or cost any money. You can do it alone or with friends, depending on your preference. And you can do it just about anywhere. To increase the intensity of your walking workout, move faster or go uphill.

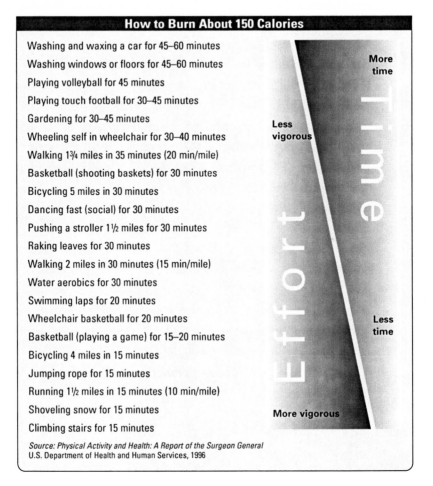

How to Burn About 150 Calories	
Washing and waxing a car for 45–60 minutes	**More time**
Washing windows or floors for 45–60 minutes	
Playing volleyball for 45 minutes	
Playing touch football for 30–45 minutes	
Gardening for 30–45 minutes	**Less vigorous**
Wheeling self in wheelchair for 30–40 minutes	
Walking 1¾ miles in 35 minutes (20 min/mile)	
Basketball (shooting baskets) for 30 minutes	
Bicycling 5 miles in 30 minutes	
Dancing fast (social) for 30 minutes	
Pushing a stroller 1½ miles for 30 minutes	
Raking leaves for 30 minutes	
Walking 2 miles in 30 minutes (15 min/mile)	
Water aerobics for 30 minutes	
Swimming laps for 20 minutes	
Wheelchair basketball for 20 minutes	**Less time**
Basketball (playing a game) for 15–20 minutes	
Bicycling 4 miles in 15 minutes	
Jumping rope for 15 minutes	
Running 1½ miles in 15 minutes (10 min/mile)	
Shoveling snow for 15 minutes	
Climbing stairs for 15 minutes	**More vigorous**

Source: Physical Activity and Health: A Report of the Surgeon General
U.S. Department of Health and Human Services, 1996

recreational activities like tennis or golf (as long as you walk the fairways); even chores like housework or yard work. Remember, the more you do the greater the health benefits you will enjoy. The benefits don't level off until you burn several thousand calories per week, something few of us are in danger of doing.

Gauging the intensity of your workouts

When taking part in any physical activity, it is important to monitor your exertion level by checking your heart rate and/or paying attention to how you feel (perceived exertion).

Heart rate: You can measure your heart rate by taking your pulse in your wrist or neck. Before exercising, sit quietly and count the heartbeats (the pulses) for fifteen seconds. Then multiply that number by four to get beats per minute. This gives you your resting heart rate (RHR). To find your exercise heart rate (EHR), exercise until you reach your regular moderate intensity and measure your pulse again. (If you can't take your pulse while moving, stop and immediately check your pulse.) Again, count heartbeats for fifteen seconds and multiply by four.

Moderate-intensity activity that is comfortably challenging is

Karvonen Formula

[(220 − age) − RHR] × % + RHR = EHR
Say you are forty years old and your RHR is 80, and you are aiming for a 50 to 75 percent exercise intensity. Fill in the numbers using the formula above, calculating it in stages:

Step 1: [(220 − age) − RHR]
[(220 − 40) − 80] = 100

Step 2: [100] × % (where the % you are aiming for is 50 to 75)
100 × 50% = 50   100 × 75% = 75

Step 3: Add RHR
50 + 80 = 130   75 + 80 = 155

Your target EHR is between 130 and 155 beats per minute.

Perceived Exertion

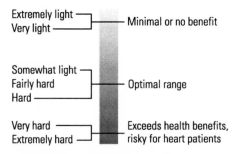

Source: Jim Huddleston, adapted from "Borg Scale of Perceived Exertion," from GA Borg: "Psychophysical Basis of Perceived Exertion," Med Sci Sports Exerc 14:377, 1982.

generally recommended for most people. It is associated with good health benefits, decreased injury risk, and enjoyment potential. Moderate to vigorous activity increases heart rate to between 50 percent and 85 percent of maximum heart rate (MHR). (A generic formula is MHR equals 220 minus your age.) For most people, aiming to increase heart rate by 50–75 percent is a reasonable goal. Even increasing your heart rate by 40 percent will provide some benefits. The Karvonen formula (see box) is a good way to calculate your target EHR. However, if you are taking heart medications such as beta-blockers or calcium channel blockers, this formula will not be accurate for you. If your doctor recommends an exercise stress test (usually on a treadmill) before you start an exercise program, you can calculate your EHR based on your performance. In this case, a true MHR can be determined from your performance instead of using the generic substitute for MHR (220 minus your age).

Perceived exertion: Another way to gauge the intensity of your exercise is to use the Borg scale, which helps you rate perceived exertion. Rather than doing a mathematical calculation, the Borg scale asks you to pay attention to how you feel.

An easy rule of thumb for determining if you are exercising at a comfortably challenging (moderate) intensity is the "talk test." You should be able to exercise and talk comfortably at the same time. For most aerobic exercise, if you have trouble talking, you are probably working too hard. (This doesn't apply for interval training, a high-intensity workout for experienced exercisers.) However, if you can sing, then you are not working hard enough. Some shortness of breath is natural. You should feel challenged, but not overwhelmed. When you finish exercising, you should feel as if you probably could have done more if necessary. Rest if you have aches, cramps, pain, fatigue, or severe shortness of breath.

The ideal approach is to use both your heart rate and perceived exertion to determine how much you should exercise at any given time. This is important not only with formal exercise, but also with activities of daily living. Be aware and use your perception of your exertion level to help pace your activities, to know when to slow down and rest or when to push a little harder.

Improving your fitness level

For total fitness, aim to achieve a good balance between aerobic fitness, flexibility, and resistance or strength training every week. As you'll discover, performing a variety of activities has benefits over doing just one type of exercise. Called cross-training, this type of exercise leads to better overall body conditioning, prevents injury, and prevents boredom, thus improving the likelihood of long-term success.

Aerobic exercise: Aerobic exercise raises heart rate and increases breathing, thereby stimulating the entire cardiovascular system. Examples include walking, swimming, bicycling, running, skating—anything that is continuous and rhythmical and gets you breathing a little harder and your heart beating faster. Aerobic exercise takes energy. Your body uses oxygen to burn fat along with blood sugar to supply

Warming Up and Cooling Down

Before and after engaging in any moderate to vigorous activity, take five to ten minutes to warm up and cool down. A warm-up and cool-down routine reduces muscle soreness, allows your heart and blood vessels to adjust to (or recover from) the increased demands of exercise, and reduces the chance of injury or muscle soreness. Both warm-up and cool-down routines provide an opportunity to become more mindful of your body, as well as to transition into and out of a more physically active state.

WARM UP

This will help prepare you for the transition from rest to exercise by increasing blood flow, respiration, and body temperature, and stretching muscles. To warm up, do a series of gentle stretches, focusing on one muscle group at a time. Hold the position for at least fifteen to twenty seconds to allow the muscle to release tension. Another good way to warm up is to do your preferred aerobic activity at a slow pace. If you want to take a brisk walk, for instance, spend five minutes walking at a slow speed to let your body ease into it. As you go through a warm-up routine, you should literally feel warmer and your body should feel more nimble and flexible.

COOL DOWN

Even more importantly, spend five to ten minutes cooling down after you complete your exercise. Although this involves much the same process as a warm-up routine, in this case the objective is to let your body gradually cool off by reducing the intensity of your movements. The cool-down period is especially important for people with heart disease. Stretching and slow movement help to:

- Increase the elasticity of your muscles
- Prevent blood from pooling in any part of your body
- Allow for a gradual dissipation of body heat and lactic acid which builds up in working muscles and can cause muscle soreness
- Reduce the chance of irregular heartbeats

that energy. Therefore aerobic exercise is a wonderful way to work toward or maintain a healthy weight while also improving your endurance and the efficiency of your cardiovascular system.

As long as you work out with the same intensity, most aerobic activities offer the same benefits. So pick the activity you enjoy most; that way you'll be more likely to do it on a regular basis. If you have a musculoskeletal condition (such as arthritis), consider swimming, walking, or working out in a pool. You will weigh less under water, and water provides support to your body, taking pressure off your bones and joints. Water also provides some resistance as you move through it, so it's a good environment for doing both weight training and aerobic exercise.

A good goal is to aim to do aerobic exercise three to five times/week for thirty to sixty minutes, but try not to miss more than two days in a row.

Exercise Safety Tips

- Drink water! Your body needs to replenish fluids lost during exercise. Drink a glass of water fifteen to thirty minutes before you exercise. On particularly hot days or when exercising longer than thirty minutes, take a drink every fifteen to twenty minutes while exercising.
- Wear proper shoes. A good supportive shoe is fine for general physical activity, but as you increase the intensity of your exercise, you may need to get sneakers designed specifically for the exercise. They're worth the investment.
- Dress smart. If exercising indoors, or in a warm environment, choose lightweight, blended fabrics that will help to wick away moisture. Cotton fabrics are not the best choice, since they absorb moisture, making you feel sticky and sweaty. In cold weather, wear several layers of light clothing: an inner layer of lightweight synthetic fabric to wick away moisture; a middle layer to provide insulation if necessary; and an outer layer that fits loosely and offers protection against the elements.

Strength training: As women age, they need weight lifting just as much as, if not more than, young people or men. This type of exercise is one of women's first lines of defense in the battle against osteoporosis. And women are stepping up to the weight machines by the millions. The fact is, strength training not only builds muscle, but also helps reduce body fat and increase bone density—a winning combination for women's health.

Contrary to myth, women are not limited to small hand weights. Women and men can follow the same program of exercises, as long as it's designed for their body size and level of strength. What you do depends on your level of ability. Some of your choices include:

- Weight machines (Nautilus, Universal, Cybex)
- Latex stretch bands
- Free weights (includes wrist and cuff weights)
- Calisthenics (sit-ups, pull-ups, push-ups, press-ups).

Strength training, sometimes called resistance or weight training or muscle toning, is an example of anaerobic exercise. You engage in short bursts of activity, such as doing sit-ups or lifting weights, that burn mostly blood sugar (glucose) to supply the energy needed for the activity. Because lifting heavy weights places sudden, intense pressure on your heart and arteries, be sure to check with your doctor before doing resistance exercises, especially if you have high blood pressure, diabetes, or heart disease. Also check with your doctor if you've ever had back problems or have osteoporosis or other musculoskeletal injuries.

Done correctly, strength training is very safe. It can also be one of the fastest workouts. Three twenty-minute sessions a week (preferably not on consecutive days), consisting of one or two sets of eight to twelve repetitions for each muscle group, will do the job.

Core strength: A growing trend in strength training is to focus on abdominal muscles and other muscles of the torso to improve posture and support the entire spine. One popular method that incorporates both strengthening and stretching is Pilates, a system of exercise involving machines and pulleys. This targets the deep abdominal muscles as well as the most visible outer layer, building a strong center or core that is crucial for a healthy, well-supported back. A modified version called Mat Pilates can be done without equipment as floor exercises. Overall, Pilates is a wonderful exercise experience for menopausal women as it helps to increase strength, balance, flexibility, and body awareness, all of which contribute to improved posture, strong backs, and fall prevention. Many gyms offer Pilates mat classes. Specialized studios have specialized equipment and provide personal training in Pilates.

Michelle, who, at age fifty-two, exercises five days a week, has worked Pilates into her cardio and strength training routine. "I could feel a physical difference in the strength of my abdominal area after three one-hour classes," she recalls. She remembers really noticing her improved endurance on a family ski trip. "By the end of the day I wasn't even tired."

Traditional abdominal strengthening exercises such as sit-ups and stretching exercises for the trunk are another option.

Flexibility and balance: Maintaining flexibility and balance through stretching exercises is the critical third leg of the exercise plan. It doesn't matter if you stretch before exercise, after, or both. Do whatever feels right for your body.

The general recommendations for stretching include:

- Do it two to three times a week.
- Hold each stretch fifteen to twenty seconds, three to five times each.
- Stretch into mild discomfort, not into pain.

Stretching is also a good time to bring an element of mindfulness into the activity. As you stretch, focus on the sensations that you feel; what's important is not how far you stretch, but how you feel as you stretch. The practices of tai chi and yoga are excellent ways to stretch and enjoy it! Both are based on Eastern philosophy and enhance balance, flexibility, relaxation, mood, vitality, and sense of well-being. These practices can stand alone as spiritual exercise experiences, or they can be incorporated into more traditional exercise to help you become more mindful and self-aware as you move and stretch.

Your Exercise Prescription

Exercise type	Duration	Frequency
Warm-up	5–10 minutes	Whenever you exercise
Aerobics	20–60 minutes	3–5 times/week
Muscle Toning	15–30 minutes	2–3 times/week
	1–2 sets of 8–12 repetitions	
Cool Down	5–10 minutes	Whenever you exercise

Take it slow and build toward these goals gradually. As you incorporate exercise into your life it won't seem so overwhelming, and you'll actually look forward to it.

Learning from Other Cultures

When it comes to broadening our perspective about exercise, we have much to learn from other cultures. In our goal-oriented Western culture, exercise is something measured by minutes, calories, and pain. Often what is lost in the process is any sense of enjoyment.

Other cultures provide a different perspective and may suggest ways to broaden your own thinking. In ancient traditions, physical activity and exercise had less of a physical focus and more of a spiritual one. The Greek philosopher Plato, for instance, regarded exercise as a

A Look at Yoga and Tai Chi

Tai chi originated in China as a form of martial arts and self-defense. It has evolved into a practice that combines movement with focused awareness in order to enable a life force known as *qi* to flow through the body. These graceful exercises relieve tension, improve balance and coordination, foster strength and flexibility, and focus the mind. This low- to moderate-intensity exercise practice improves cardiovascular health, bolsters immune system function, increases flexibility and strength, and decreases risk of falls. In a randomized, controlled study measuring frailty and injuries, tai chi was found to:

- Reduce the onset of falls by 47.5 percent
- Reduce the fear of falling
- Increase participants' confidence in taking part in activities

Yoga is a spiritual exercise practice that enables you to develop and maintain musculoskeletal health by realigning your posture, releasing tension, improving balance, and increasing flexibility, while also helping to cultivate mind/body awareness. Movement into and out of yoga postures provides the necessary weight-bearing stress to stimulate bone and cartilage health and the movement to stretch and tone muscles.

means of developing the spiritual side of life. According to the Vedic text of Buddhism, the main purpose of exercise was to rejuvenate the body and cultivate the mind, developing mind/body coordination.

Even today, many cultures use physical activity as a way to celebrate history and community. In Africa dance is often used to celebrate life, culture, and generate healing. In the African healing dance, dancers mimic the movements of animals and nature to connect with the world and draw healing energy from it. Similarly, Native American people in this country have long used dances for ceremony, story telling, and entertainment, not just exercise. Yoga originated in India and tai chi in China, but both have become very popular in the United

Lighten Your Mental Load by Moving Some Heavy Weight

One way to exercise your soul as well as your body is by lifting weights and following these guidelines (for more details on strength training, see pages 132–33):

- Focus on your breath, your form, and the sensation of your muscles while lifting the weight.
- Move the weight slowly in the rhythm of your breath. Breathe out as you lift the weight, breathe in as you return to the starting position.
- Pay attention to how your body feels, not to negative thoughts telling you to hurry up or lift more weight.
- When you do increase the weights, watch your form to avoid injury.
- Let go of distracting thoughts and bring awareness back to the breath.

States and can be considered as much a philosophy as a physical practice.

Embracing Mindfulness in Exercise

A component of a truly spiritual workout is mindfulness. As discussed in Chapter 3, mindfulness is the ability to focus on only the thing you are currently doing (in this case, exercise). An example of mindfulness would be to focus on the cadence of your strokes and the rhythm of your breaths during a swim. Really feel the cool water breaking at the tips of your fingers. Then pay attention to the way in which each muscle moves to propel the body through the cool liquid. Truly enjoying what you are doing is part of the process.

Another way to incorporate mindfulness into exercise is to try mindful walking. During a mindful walk, you are not thinking about what you will be doing when you finish your walk, or what you think you should be doing instead of taking this time for yourself. And the activity doesn't have to have a particular goal. Mindful walking is not just about getting to a destination; it's also about the experiences you have and what you learn about yourself while getting there. It is about process rather than outcome. As Robert Louis Stevenson once said, "To travel hopefully is a better thing than to arrive."

Mindful walking satisfies the body's need to exercise and the soul's need to relax and reflect. It represents the coexistence of inner silence and outer activity. As such, mindful walking is exercise for the whole person. Similar in philosophy to yoga, mindful walking involves every part of us: mind, body, and spirit (or soul).

The best approach to mindful walking is the one that works for you. Be flexible and open to all possibilities. No matter which technique you use, it is likely that your attention will drift at times. Just acknowledge the distracting thoughts, much as you would clouds in the sky, and then refocus. Here are some tips on how to walk mindfully:

- Focus on your breathing. Breathe deeply through your nose. Breathe in the good (energy, awareness, love, peace, serenity) and breathe out the bad (frustrations, distractions, fear, pain).
- Pay attention to the cadence of your steps as you walk. Steps are a physical mantra. Try to time the rhythm of your breath with the rhythm of your steps. Count to four slowly as you breathe inward, matching each number with a step, and to four again as you exhale.
- Add a mantra or some type of affirmation to your cadence. A three-count cadence (similar to the waltz) is slightly less rhythmical than a four-count cadence, and thus may hold your attention more. Some examples of three-count cadences:

I am here
I can walk
I am strong

- Attend to nature. Delight in the beauty of the world around you and let your natural rhythm flow with the rhythm of nature.
- You can also add spiritual or religious elements so that your mindful walk becomes a prayer walk.

Overcoming Barriers

You know it's good for you and it'll make you feel better, so why is it hard to get moving and commit to regular exercise? Ask people about exercise, and often what you get are complaints. Some people find health clubs intimidating, others say they feel too tired to exercise, still others don't like to sweat. You may be among those overwhelmed at the thought of starting to exercise after a lifetime of sedentary living. The biggest complaint we hear, though, is lack of

One Woman's Story

As the pressures of the day mount, exercise serves as a release for many people. For one of the women in our program who's busy with a job and two teenage children, there comes a time when she must walk away from it all, literally. "I say I need time out and I leave and go take a walk. I even do some short bursts of running." Tina says. "When I start to run, all the stress begins to dissipate."

Tina's response to stress is one of the healthiest. And her introduction to exercise-induced relaxation response (RR) came about by accident. Her love of swimming could put her into a state of deep relaxation, but she didn't recognize what was happening until talking to one of our group leaders. Today, she regularly combines swimming and the RR for a workout that benefits her mind and body: "I go swimming for twenty minutes and it's like I'm addicted. I just feel so great when I get out of the pool. It totally clears my head and it changes my breathing pattern. It just slows everything right down. I'm exercising and my heart is pumping, but it completely clears my head and I feel exhilarated when I'm done."

time. Internal barriers exist because we allow them to. Challenge your assumptions. Lack of time, for instance, should not be a factor on a regular basis.

Make time: In a sixteen-hour day, surely there are thirty minutes you can spend on physical activity, especially when you can break it down into three ten-minute segments. Set up a reasonable plan that you can fit into your schedule. Think it through. You may need to give something up (a half hour of TV or sleep, for example) to fit in your workout. Try to pick the time of day that works best for you, and have a backup plan for bad weather (if you exercise outdoors) or for those very hectic days.

If you feel plagued by to-do lists and lack of time, remember that exercise can help pull you away from emotions like anger or stress, and you may find your productivity after the workout more than makes up for the half hour you spent.

Challenge negative thoughts: If you have a knee-jerk negative reaction to exercise, think about why. What thoughts prevent you from being open to a new type of activity?

Set reasonable goals: Behavior change takes time, so start slowly and build gradually. Do not attempt any physical activity that feels more demanding than you can handle. Set reasonable goals and enjoy the journey of reaching them.

Rethink success: Often we approach exercise with a kind of all-or-nothing thinking. But it's normal to make progress, then get off track for a while, then start exercising again. Every step you take is a step in the right direction. Support helps, so seek company. Walking with a friend can provide the encouragement you need at the beginning.

Aim for a lifetime of physical activity, and if you find yourself slipping from your exercise habit, instead of beating yourself up about it, look at it as a learning experience. What happened? Why did you stop exercising? What got in the way? Can you prevent it from happening again? The answers to these questions will help you get back on track and stay there.

Find joy in the process: Although goals are important, so is enjoying yourself. Focus more on the process of an activity, rather than the outcome. Once you have set your goals, let them go and instead focus on the experiences you have while getting there. As the philosopher Alan Watts once said, "You don't dance to get to the other side of the floor."

Success with exercise comes with the realization that exercise isn't just about burning calories or getting your heart rate to a certain level. It really is about self-nurture, appreciating yourself as a physical, emotional, and spiritual being, and doing what you can to maximize your mind/body health. So use the tools and advice we have provided in this chapter to develop a rhythm of physical activity that fits into your life. When you make physical activity an integral part of who you are, you have taken a big step toward living a healthier, happier life.

CHAPTER 6

Nutrition: The Healing Plate

Women repeatedly tell us that changing the foods they eat has made a big difference in how they feel. You've heard "good" food is "good" medicine. Well, it's true. Foods rich in nutrients, antioxidants, calcium, and essential oils can help us feel better, think better, build bone, and reduce risk for heart disease and cancer. On the other hand, a poor diet can sap our energy and truly make us feel lousy.

We'll begin with some nutrition basics that should help you get the nutrients you need for general health and well-being and to maintain your energy. We'll then discuss the foods that can help manage menopausal symptoms.

The Balanced Plate

One major problem in this country has been a model of eating that is outdated and damaging. We have relied too heavily on artery-clogging saturated fats and refined carbohydrates and we are paying for it in the form of illness and fatigue. At midlife, women are more vulnerable to heart disease, osteoporosis, and feelings of fatigue. One of the best ways to counter these health problems is to balance your plate. Many of our patients find that the balanced plate is one of the most effective tools and an easy approach for lowering cholesterol and blood pressure, losing weight, and improving the way they feel.

When you look at the typical American's plate, you often find a huge piece of meat, poultry, or fish occupying most of the plate, with generous helpings of white bread, potatoes, or white rice on the side. At other times, the entire plate is filled with white pasta, which is high in calories and carbohydrates, completely lacking in nutrients, and digested so quickly that you soon find yourself hungry again. Vegetables and fruits, if they are on the plate at all, are added as an afterthought.

The typical American plate (see top and bottom left illustrations on page 143) is an unbalanced meal that is high in calories and saturated fat, low in essential nutrients that fight chronic disease, and dominated by the type of carbohydrates that are not good in large amounts. By eating from this plate, you are not only increasing your risk of heart disease (or worsening it) but also increasing your risk for other chronic diseases such as cancer.

To balance your plate and reduce your risk for disease, start by filling half of your plate with vegetables. Then fill one-fourth with a source of protein, and the remaining fourth with whole grains or some other type of healthy starch, such as brown rice or whole wheat bread (see top and bottom right illustrations on page 143).

The beauty of this approach is that it is easy to implement, even for busy people. What's great is you don't have to take time to measure food with this strategy. The plate serves as a guide.

Benefits of the balanced plate

With a balanced plate, you achieve four important health goals.

1. Reduce total calories, since vegetables average only about 25 calories per serving (about one-third of the calories of protein foods and starches), which can help with body fat loss.

2. Increase your intake of vital nutrients, such as antioxidants, B vitamins, phytochemicals from various plant sources, and fiber, all of which are important for good health.
3. Reduce your intake of saturated fat, which will improve your cholesterol levels and help to prevent heart disease.
4. Reduce your consumption of carbohydrates, which helps weight loss and helps to prevent insulin resistance and diabetes.

Quantity and quality

Choosing healthy portions is important but filling those portions with healthy foods is another challenge. Limiting hidden fats, starches, and calories can help prevent chronic diseases.

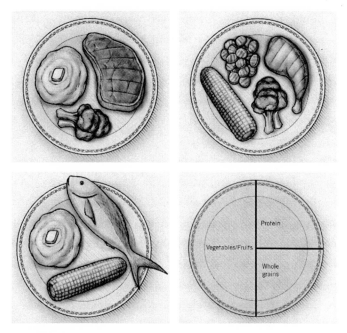

Balancing Your Plate

The meat-and-starch-heavy plate (top left) and the starch-heavy plate (bottom left) should be avoided. Picture a plate divided into three sections: one-half should be for vegetables, one-fourth for healthy protein, and one-fourth for healthy carbohydrates (bottom right). This can be done without sacrificing taste (top right).

Know your vegetables: Not all vegetables are created equal. You know this if you've ever been famished and had to choose between green beans and a potato as a side dish. Chances are, you chose the potato. When balancing a plate, consider this: some vegetables act as hidden starches. While most vegetables have 25 calories and 5 grams of carbohydrates per serving, five vegetables—*corn, peas, potatoes, sweet potatoes,* and *winter squash*—have about 80 calories and triple the amount of carbohydrates per serving. Beans require some thought as well. Green beans are the only type of beans low in calories and starch. All others are roughly half starch and half protein. That's why the bottom left plate in the illustration should be avoided: It's loaded with these hidden starches (corn *and* potatoes).

If you find it too difficult to create a plate that is half full of vegetables, compromise by dividing your plate into thirds, so that vegetables, protein, and starch are present in equal portions. This type of plate is still better than the typical American plate. Whatever you do, try to work more vegetables into your meals. Dividing the plate into thirds—fruit, protein, and a whole grain starch—is good for breakfast, too.

"Hidden" starches: We recommend substituting starchy vegetables for white rice, white bread, and other refined starches. If you enjoy corn on the cob, for instance, substitute this vegetable for rice or pasta when making up a balanced plate. Beans provide additional flexibility, because you can treat them as starch or protein when building a balanced plate. If you eat beans with a protein source such as chicken, treat the beans as a starch (so if you mix them with rice, the mixture should still take up only one-fourth of your plate). If you are having a vegetarian meal of beans and rice, treat the beans as protein (so half your plate would be beans and rice, while the other half should be filled with low calorie vegetables such as tomatoes, summer squash, and salad).

Pick your protein: Most protein foods deliver more than just protein itself, so it's important to consider the big picture as you create a balanced plate. First of all, the portion should be about the size of a deck of playing cards or at the absolute maximum one and a half decks. Proteins high in saturated fats tend to clog arteries, so limit your intake of full-fat dairy products and red meats.

Red meat: Because red meat is so high in saturated fats, limit your intake to once or twice a week. Beef, lamb, veal, and pork are all considered red meat (except for pork tenderloin—treat pork tenderloin like poultry). You can reduce the fat you eat by buying cuts with the word "round" in them. The next leanest cuts are the loins. Buy ground beef that is at least 90 percent fat free.

Poultry: Chicken, turkey, and game hens are generally better choices than red meat, but only if you pay attention to what you're eating. Choose white meat over dark meat. If you choose ground turkey, read the label to make sure the skin is not ground in (skin adds saturated fat and doubles the calories).

Seafood: Fatty fish, low-fat fish, and shellfish are all good choices. Seafood is heart-healthy because it is low in, and sometimes completely free of, saturated fat. The fats in some fatty fish, such as salmon and sardines, provide heart-healthy omega-3 oils. But even low-fat fish with negligible amounts of omega-3 fats are healthy.

Beans: Beans (including soy products), as mentioned, can work as either a protein or a starch. They are a great choice for protein because they are low in fat but high in fiber, minerals, and vitamins.

Soy: Some soy products make excellent substitutions for meat at meals. If you've never eaten soy before, start with a soy veggie burger.

Eggs: They are not just for breakfast anymore. One to two hardboiled eggs later in the day can provide a great source of protein on a lunch salad or as a snack. If you need to limit cholesterol but keep the protein, choose the egg substitutes or eat only the egg white.

Dairy products: Milk, cheese, yogurt, and cottage cheese all have moderate amounts of protein. Try to stick to low-fat versions, since the predominant type of fat in all of them is the artery-clogging saturated fats. Be aware that milk and yogurts are not only moderate sources of protein but they also contain carbohydrates naturally.

Nuts, seeds, and nut butters: All three of these are high in protein, healthy fats, and fiber, but they are also high in calories. So include them with meals or snacks regularly, but limit portions to one-quarter cup of nuts or seeds and two tablespoons of nut butters.

Fruit: Fruits and vegetables are often lumped together when it comes to dietary advice, but we recommend that you treat them separately. Fruits are loaded with nutrients, phytochemicals, antioxidants, and fiber, but they also contain natural sugars. This means they contain more calories than vegetables (fruit averages 60 calories per serving) and if you eat fruits too often, or several at once, your blood sugar levels and triglycerides may rise. Eat two to four servings a day of fresh fruit, canned fruits without any syrup, dried fruits, or juice (no more than 4–6 fl. oz. daily), but spread your fruit intake throughout the day.

When it comes to food, the healthiest approach is to emulate birds: eat small meals throughout the day. Instead of the traditional three-meals-a-day approach, try reducing plate size (and portions) at breakfast, lunch, and dinner, then add one or two healthy snacks in between regular meals or at night. As long as your plate is balanced, this approach will help keep your blood sugar levels stable and supply your body with a steady stream of energy.

Steady Your Blood Sugar: Monitoring Your Carbohydrates

Kelly's day started off with coffee and a bagel. Within a few hours she would feel fatigued. But her life was busy. To boost her energy, she would reach for something quick and easy—four cookies and a handful of pretzels. She'd feel good for an hour but the cycle would continue and she'd feel fatigued again soon after.

If this sounds familiar, you may be experiencing what has been described as a blood sugar roller coaster, induced by too many starchy carbohydrates. The problem is not carbohydrates. Complex carbohydrates like whole grains and beans are an essential part of any diet. The problem is the overabundance of processed carbohydrates like refined white breads and pastas in our diets. These processed foods break down too easily in the body. They are then quickly converted into sugar and eventually stored as fat.

The blood sugar roller coaster

Think of carbohydrates from the perspective of your digestive tract, which transforms what we eat into energy our bodies can use. When you digest food, all carbohydrates (including starches, which are long chains of sugars) break down into sugar that can enter the bloodstream, but some break down more quickly than others do. That's why most dietitians today talk about carbohydrates in terms of their "glycemic index," the rate at which blood sugar rises after you eat. Carbohydrates with a high glycemic index, such as white bread and potatoes, create a spike in blood sugar that, in turn, triggers a surge of insulin. Insulin enables the body to take sugar out of the blood and give it to the cells to either burn it as energy or convert it into fat for storage. As your insulin levels spike to take the sugar out of the blood, your blood sugar levels plummet, making you feel hungry so that you will want to eat again.

Many dietitians now believe that one of the reasons Americans have grown so fat is that they are overeating the wrong type of carbohydrates (often with the best of intentions, to reduce fat consumption) and have unwittingly become riders on the blood sugar roller coaster. Ride the blood sugar roller coaster too often, and you may develop insulin resistance, so that tissues in your body become deaf to insulin's call to absorb sugar, and blood sugar levels remain abnormally high.

This can lead to *Syndrome X*. As discussed in Chapter 5, this metabolic syndrome usually involves having abdominal obesity, diabetes, borderline or high blood pressure, elevated cholesterol, and elevated triglycerides. One study estimated that Syndrome X doubles the risk of high blood pressure and triples the risk of heart disease.

Get off the roller coaster

To get off the blood sugar roller coaster, eat healthy carbohydrates such as whole grain products, dried beans, and vegetables. These foods tend to be digested more slowly, so that blood sugar levels rise and ebb more slowly, exerting a similar calming effect on insulin levels. This will help you feel satisfied longer while obtaining more nutrients and vitamins.

To get smart when it comes to starch, reduce your consumption of refined foods, especially products made of white flour, and instead get rough: eat more whole grain products and vegetables. You will get even better satiation if you combine whole grains with an unsaturated fat (for example, olive oil) or some protein.

By keeping your blood sugar levels modulated, you will also find that you are in a better mood, think more clearly, perform better at work, and are able to maintain your energy levels throughout the day. That mid-afternoon fog that so many people experience after eating lunch will be a memory once you substitute healthy carbohydrates for those that are highly refined and balance them with a protein source or unsaturated fat.

Healthy Snack Suggestions

To create a healthy snack, try one of the following combinations. Or make up your own, by pairing a source of protein or healthy fat with a carbohydrate.

Protein Source	Carbohydrates
natural peanut butter (1 Tbsp), with	whole grain bread
1% or skim milk, with	whole grain cereal
low-fat or fat-free yogurt, with	fruit/Grapenuts
bean dip or hummus, with	whole grain crackers
cheese (low fat), with	whole grain crackers
nuts (¼ cup or less), with	dried fruits (2 tablespoons)

For Kelly, correcting the "carbo" coaster meant planning ahead by bringing snacks with her that were balanced and more satisfying, like nuts with fruit. Satisfying snacks can be hard to find in the middle of the day if you're on the move because they're not readily available at convenience stores or coffee shops. Best bet: carry a zip-lock bag with a protein and whole grain snack.

Fiber

Fiber comes in two varieties. Insoluble fiber satisfies hunger pangs and helps to regulate bowel movements, and it may reduce your risk of colon cancer. It also helps prevent diverticular disease and constipation. Soluble fiber reduces cholesterol and triglyceride levels by about 10 percent, and may help to regulate blood sugar.

Whole grain sources of insoluble fiber include brown rice, whole wheat bread, and whole grain cereals or pasta. Make sure the word "whole" is on the list of ingredients. Many so-called health products list "wheat flour," which is just another name for refined white flour.

Major Sources of Fiber

Soluble	Insoluble
oat bran	wheat bran
oatmeal	whole wheat flour
legumes	whole grains (breads, cereals, etc.)
apples	vegetables
barley	fruits
carrots	psyllium*
psyllium*	

* Found in supplements such as Metamucil and in Bran Buds cereal

Whenever possible, substitute whole grain products for white rice, white bread, and fiber-free cereals such as Corn Flakes or Rice Krispies. You can also "think outside the rice box" by trying grains like kasha, bulgur, quinoa, and couscous.

To consume adequate amounts of fiber, choose cereals that have at least *three grams of fiber per serving* and try to eat other fiber-rich foods throughout the day. It is often best to add fiber gradually, while drinking plenty of water. Talk to your clinician about ways to boost your fiber intake, including whether or not fiber supplements are right for you.

Dietary Fats: Friends and Foes

Suffice it to say that decades of research now show that fats can be friends as well as foes. Over the years, we have learned that dietary fat does not necessarily make us fat. In fact, "good" fats reduce our risk for heart disease. To understand the role of fat, think of your body as a factory. What you consume serves as the raw material that produces the energy that moves your muscles, fuels your brain, and

The new healthy eating pyramid

Type of food	Healthy eating recommendations (per day)
Fats & sweets	• Use olive, soy, corn, sunflower, or peanut oils • Limit saturated fats and trans ("hydrogenated") fats • Limit sweets
Dairy products	• 1–2 servings of low-fat dairy products, a daily calcium supplement, or both
Meat, poultry, fish, eggs, nuts, & legumes	• 1–3 servings of nuts and legumes • 0–2 servings fish, poultry, or eggs • Choose vegetable sources of protein, such as nuts and beans, more often than animal sources, such as red meat and dairy products
Vegetables & fruits	• 5 or more servings of vegetables • 2–3 servings of fruit
Bread, cereal, pasta, & rice	• Eat whole grains and whole-grain products liberally • Limit potatoes and refined carbohydrates such as white bread, white rice, and pasta
Multivitamin	• Take one a day

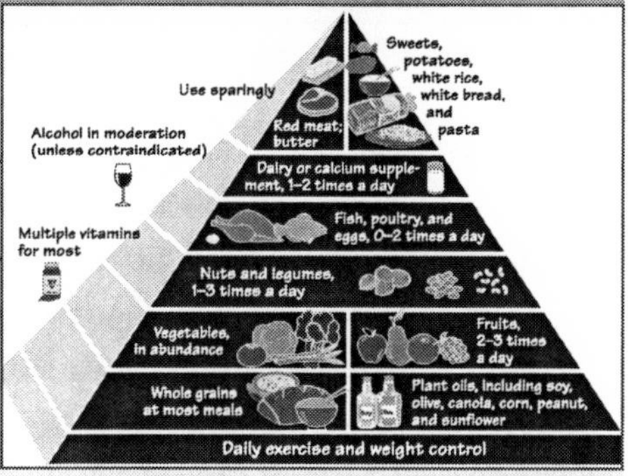
Sweets, potatoes, white rice, white bread, and pasta
Use sparingly
Red meat; butter
Alcohol in moderation (unless contraindicated)
Dairy or calcium supplement, 1–2 times a day
Multiple vitamins for most
Fish, poultry, and eggs, 0–2 times a day
Nuts and legumes, 1–3 times a day
Vegetables, in abundance
Fruits, 2–3 times a day
Whole grains at most meals
Plant oils, including soy, olive, canola, corn, peanut, and sunflower
Daily exercise and weight control

Serving sense

One serving of dairy products equals:
- 1 cup milk or yogurt
- $1\frac{1}{2}$ ounces natural cheese

One serving of meat, poultry, fish, dry beans, eggs, or nuts equals:
- 2–3 ounces cooked lean meat, poultry, or fish
- $1–1\frac{1}{2}$ cups cooked dry beans
- 2–3 eggs
- 4–6 tablespoons peanut butter

One serving of vegetables or fruit equals:
- 1 cup raw, leafy vegetables
- $\frac{1}{2}$ cup of other vegetables or fruit, cooked or chopped
- 1 medium banana or orange
- $\frac{1}{2}$ cup fruit or vegetable juice

One serving of bread, cereal, rice, or pasta equals:
- 1 slice bread
- 1 ounce ready-to-eat cereal
- $\frac{1}{2}$ cup cooked cereal, rice, or pasta

Adapted from *Eat, Drink, and Be Healthy: The Harvard Medical School Guide to Healthy Eating* by Dr. Walter Willett (Simon & Schuster, 2001).

The Healthy Eating Pyramid created by Dr. Walter Willett is set up to recommend a low glycemic diet that is nutrient dense. We recommend this pyramid because it presents a healthier diet than the original Food Guide Pyramid. For more details about the Healthy Eating Pyramid read Dr. Willett's *Eat, Drink, and Be Healthy.*

keeps cells functioning properly. And "good" fats, like oil for machinery, are essential in keeping the operation running smoothly.

Healthy fats

The *unsaturated* fats—monounsaturated and polyunsaturated—are particularly healthy for your heart. Unsaturated fats lower both total and harmful LDL cholesterol. Vary your sources to ensure a good mixture of both, paying special attention to foods rich in the omega-3 polyunsaturated fats (see table on page 153). These are essential fatty acids your body can't make on its own.

Monounsaturated fats: In the 1990s, many experts touted monounsaturated fats as the best choice because they maintained levels of helpful high density lipoprotein HDL ("good" cholesterol), but the emerging consensus is that polyunsaturated fats also do this provided they are consumed in the right amounts. Still, monounsaturated fat found in foods like olive oil, peanuts and peanut oil, avocados, and almonds is an excellent source of healthy fats.

Polyunsaturated fats: Polyunsaturated fats appear to lower total cholesterol more than monounsaturated fats. Polyunsaturated fats are easy to find in the American diet. They come in the form of vegetable oils (sunflower, sesame, corn, safflower, and soybean), as well as in nuts like walnuts, cashews, and pistachios. To increase these fats in your diet, use the oils in cooking and salad dressing. Nuts are good snacks in moderation.

Omega-3 fats: Your body cannot produce omega-3 fats, so they are classified as *essential fatty acids* and are needed to fuel fundamental cellular processes, maintain skin quality, and improve overall immunity.

Consuming sufficient amounts of omega-3 fats can be difficult since they are found only in a limited number of foods like fatty fish, walnuts, flaxseeds, and canola oil. Nevertheless, try to eat a serving or two every day. Just remember, the serving sizes are small.

Flaxseeds contain five times the essential fats of any other nut, seed, or oil. These very flat and tiny brown seeds are found in health food stores. Grind them in a hand-held coffee grinder to maximize absorption in the intestines. Sprinkle on cereal, yogurts, salads, or in homemade shakes. (Refrigerate leftovers.) If you don't grind them, you risk swallowing most of them whole and having them pass through your body without much digestion or absorption.

Flaxseeds also contain phytochemicals (substances found in plants) called lignans that may help to reduce hot flashes. Margot tried crushing whole flaxseeds and sprinkling them on her cereal each morning to see if they could help her reduce hot flashes. After a few weeks she noticed the hot flashes had dissipated. The next time she went to the store she went for convenience and bought pre-crushed flaxseed. In the following weeks her hot flashes returned, until she went back to crushing them herself. She attributed the freshness of crushing the seeds just before eating them to higher amounts of active isoflavones.

Choose fresh flaxseeds over flaxseed oils since the shell of the seed protects the oil inside the shell from oxidation. This is important since flaxseed oil can become rancid quicker than most oils. If you're going to choose flaxseed oil rather than fresh flaxseeds, be sure you buy one that contains lignans, which are the natural isoflavones, and store it in your refrigerator.

Food Sources of Omega-3 Fatty Acids

• Fatty fish (salmon; mackerel; blue fish; lake trout; swordfish; sardines; yellow fin or blue fin tuna)	• 3 to 5 ounces, one to three times per week. Canned fish contains large amounts of sodium; if possible, choose fresh fish.
• Flaxseeds	• 1 to 2 tablespoons per day
• Walnuts	• 2 to 4 tablespoons per day
• Canola oil	• 2 teaspoons to 1 tablespoon per day
• Soybean oil (vegetable oil)	• 2 teaspoons to 1 tablespoon per day

The Word on Nuts

Nuts and seeds contain a lot of nutrients in a small package. Just remember they are high in calories, so portion control is important. Limit quantities to one-quarter cup or less without shells. The best way to incorporate them into a meal is to sprinkle two to four tablespoons on cereal, yogurt, salads, or on stir-fried food. They are also great as protein-packed snacks.

Unhealthy fats

Both saturated fats and "trans" fats are harmful to the heart. While it may be impossible to avoid these fats completely, you should try to reduce consumption as much as possible. Whenever you are able, choose one of the healthier fats we've just described.

Saturated fats: Theoretically, we don't even need to consume saturated fat, since our body can make its own supply. Consuming saturated fat in your diet increases your cholesterol levels and can lead to clogged arteries, but some saturated fats are worse than others. Those contained in butter and whole-milk dairy products are the worst in terms of raising levels of harmful LDL cholesterol. Those in red meats and other beef products boost LDL slightly less. (Some good news: chocolate boosts LDL the least of all saturated fats. That means you can occasionally indulge in a chocolate or two; just don't overdo it.) While most liquid oils contain a mixture of saturated, monounsaturated, and polyunsaturated fats, try to avoid the so-called tropical oils (those from tropical lands, such as palm oil and coconut oil), which contain the largest percentage of saturated fats.

"Trans" or hydrogenated fats: These are essentially man-made saturated fats, but in some ways are even worse. Trans fats are made by taking a liquid unsaturated oil and bubbling hydrogen gas through it to make the fat hard at room temperature. Not only are these fats bad for your heart, but also recent studies have concluded that they may increase your risk of cancer. The prestigious Institute of Medicine recently concluded that there is *no safe level* of trans fat in the diet and recommended that people consume as little as possible.

Unfortunately, that won't be easy. First of all, trans fats are abundant in the typical American diet. The largest source of trans fats is deep fried restaurant foods, such as fried seafood platters, fried chicken, french fries, and doughnuts. Trans fats are also found in many packaged baked good (breads, crackers, cookies), as well as peanut butter that does not have liquid oil on top.

If trans fats are so bad, why are they so prevalent in restaurants and grocery stores? The simple answer: money. Food manufacturers continue to use trans fats because they are inexpensive, extend the shelf life of foods, and make food crispy. They are often used in restaurants because they have a high smoking point, which makes them great for deep frying food.

In 2002, a report from the National Institute of Medicine nudged the Food and Drug Administration to move ahead with its long-stalled plans to force food companies to list trans fats along with saturated fats. The FDA will begin enforcing this policy in January 2006. Until packages can catch up with the requirement, read labels carefully. Here are some tips.

Picking a margarine: Softer margarines, such as tub or semiliquid margarines, usually have less trans fats than harder stick margarines. Some types, like Promise and Smart Balance, don't contain any trans fats. Other "trans-free" brands contain less than half a gram per serving.

Eating out: Go easy on deep-fried foods. Many restaurants now use hydrogenated vegetable oils in their deep fryers. Foods fried this way can be advertised as "cholesterol free" and "cooked in vegetable oil." Even so, they can deliver a wallop of trans fats.

At the grocery store: Many prepared foods, from cookies and crackers to breaded fish sticks and frozen pot pies, contain trans fats. Right now, you have to squint at the tiny print in the ingredients list for hydrogenated, margarine, shortening, or partially hydrogenated oil. The higher these are on the list, the more trans fat the food contains.

At home: Using olive oil or canola oil for frying is a simple way to avoid trans fats. Baking can be a bit trickier. Try to avoid prepared mixes, and use trans-free margarines whenever possible.

Managing Cholesterol Levels

Type of Blood Lipid	Ideal	Ways to Get There
Total cholesterol	Less than 200	Reduce intake of saturated and trans fats
LDL (unhealthy cholesterol)	Less than 130 for women without coronary artery disease; less than 100 for women with coronary artery disease	Reduce intake of saturated and trans fats
HDL (healthy cholesterol)	More than 40	Exercise more Lose weight Stop smoking
Triglycerides	Less than 150	Reduce carbohydrate intake (starches and sugars) Reduce total fat intake Reduce alcohol intake Eat more fatty fish or flaxseeds

B vitamins: Three B vitamins in particular—B_6, B_{12}, and folic acid—appear to protect against heart disease, probably because they reduce levels of homocysteine, a by-product made as your body digests and metabolizes protein. High levels of homocysteine damage artery walls and may increase the risk of heart disease. In the Nurses' Health Study, it was reported that the risk of heart disease was reduced in the women who took a multivitamin (which was the biggest source of folate and B_6 in the study). You can usually obtain the recommended levels by taking a daily multivitamin or eating fortified breakfast cereals.

Nutrition and Menopausal Symptoms

The idea of healing through food rather than medicine is appealing to women who are experiencing menopause symptoms, but are wary of potential side effects of pharmaceuticals.

The food-mood roller coaster

There are many reasons we reach for "junk" foods—cravings, stress, fatigue, loneliness, anger, and depression. And, it's not all about a loss of willpower. There are biochemical reasons you may be reaching for chocolate or that bag of chips. One of the brain chemicals that make us feel good is serotonin. When you eat a high carbohydrate food (sweets or starches) a larger amount of tryptophan, an amino acid in your blood, is able to reach the brain. Since serotonin is produced using tryptophan, a large amount of serotonin can be produced in the brain, which improves mood and helps to curb cravings. But, just as it can affect your blood sugar and energy levels, it can also have a roller-coaster effect on your mood.

In some cases, sweets appear to trigger fatigue and feelings of depression. If a sugary food is used to raise serotonin levels, you may feel better for a short period of time, but the feelings of fatigue and depression will return soon after eating. The slump prompts you to reach for another sugary food, leading to a vicious cycle. A better option would be to eat a whole grain starch with each meal and snack to help maintain serotonin levels for longer periods of time.

Dieting and cravings: Ever wonder why you can't seem to lose weight, or why yo-yo dieting can be such a problem? Our bodies were made to resist weight loss so that we could, if the situation arose, survive a famine. That doesn't seem to be a problem for most of us nowadays. But dieting can mimic famine, triggering an inborn survival mechanism: a brain chemical called galanin. When we follow a very low calorie diet (like some current high protein diets), the body begins to break down fat tissue. The brain notices the fat breakdown and releases galanin, which causes a craving for fatty foods (often junk foods).

Crash dieting, by skipping meals or drastically reducing your calorie intake, may not only cause fatty food cravings but it also can slow the amount of calories you burn. Confronted with a sudden and severe reduction in calories, your body reacts as if you were starving and begins to conserve energy. Metabolism slows by as much as 45 percent. This means no additional weight is lost even though you reduce calorie intake. This is great if you actually are in a situation where food is scarce, not so good if you are trying to lose weight.

Interestingly, stress and PMS can also stimulate galanin release. This could partly explain why women have cravings during these times.

Soy and hot flashes

The search for healthy and healing solutions is, at least partially, responsible for the growing popularity of soy products in the United

States. Once considered odd foods found in health food stores, soy products now take premiere shelf space at conventional supermarkets in the forms of soy dogs, veggie burgers, and many other favorites. Soy products can help reduce the risk of heart disease when combined with a diet low in saturated fat and cholesterol. The question many women have is "Can soy help me manage hot flashes?"

While anecdotal stories of soy abound, clinical studies have been inconclusive as to its effectiveness in controlling hot flashes. In dietary studies of whole foods, large amounts of soy appeared to reduce the number of hot flashes. But other studies have been contradictory. Varying dosages may be part of the reason for this. We suggest eating whole foods if you want to incorporate soy into your diet. Soy protein powders are acceptable, but talk with your clinician. And, we strongly advise against taking pills. The problem with pills is that they could be giving you doses that rival a pharmaceutical dosage. And there's a lot we don't know about the effects of phytoestrogens (plant chemicals that act like estrogen in the body).

There are upwards of twenty compounds classified as phytoestrogens. Soy and flaxseed outdistance the rest in terms of phytoestrogen content, including isoflavones. Isoflavones are the natural compounds in soy and other plants that can produce estrogen-like effects in the human body. But there are differences between natural human estrogen sources and these plant-derived compounds.

When a woman's natural estrogen links to an estrogen receptor, it changes the receptor's shape, and the receptor's transformation initiates a series of reactions. During this interaction, human estrogen links to two types of estrogen receptors—alpha and beta. The phytoestrogens of plants, on the other hand, may link to only one or the other. Depending on which receptor they bind to, they may have the same effect as estrogen or they may act like an anti-estrogen, linking to the receptor, but failing to initiate the necessary reaction. In the latter case, they just sit there, blocking estrogen's access to the receptor.

When there is a lot of estrogen circulating in the body, phyto-estrogens tend to have an anti-estrogen effect. When there are lower amounts of estrogen circulating in the body, phytoestrogens tend to have a mild pro-estrogen effect (meaning they act like estrogen in the body). The key point is that phytoestrogens can alter the effects of estrogen in the body.

While there is concern about estrogenic effects on the breast and breast cancer, phytoestrogens are weaker than human estrogens. They are broken down in the body more readily and are not stored in fat. Thus, they are associated with fewer side effects. And in the form of food, phytoestrogens would likely pose few if any problems. But their effect on the breast remains unclear.

Soy's effects on breast tissue: Soy is the only phytoestrogen-containing food that has been widely studied for its effects on breast tissue. But the estrogenic and anti-estrogenic properties of soy continue to evade a strong conclusion on its ultimate effects. On one hand, observational studies have consistently shown the nations with the highest consumption of phytoestrogens have the lowest rates of breast cancer. On the other hand, several experiments have shown that soy proteins cause breast-cancer cells to proliferate.

One explanation for this (which is also an explanation of the role of hormone therapy in the development of breast cancer) is that soy proteins may promote but not initiate breast tumors. In other words, they may fan the flames but they don't start the fire. Another is that the proteins extracted from soy for use in lab experiments are not representative of soybeans in the diet because some nutrients, which may contribute to soy's protective effect, are eliminated. Obviously, a

Large Sources of Soy Protein with Isoflavones

Products	Serving Size	Soy Protein	Isoflavones
Soy protein shakes	2 scoops	20 g	55 mg
Nutlettes soy cereal	½ cup	20 g	122 mg
Soy rocks	1.25 ounces	10 g	45 mg
Soybean nuts	¼ cup	10 g	60 mg
Soy butter	2 tablespoons	8 g	38 mg
Tempeh	4 ounces	11–16 g	40 mg
Edamame (fresh soybeans)	½ cup	6–9 g	35 mg
Soy flour	¼ cup	15 g	73 mg

great deal of additional research is required for a better understanding of the role of phytoestrogens in breast cancer. For more information about soy and hot flashes, see Chapter 8.

Strong bones from soy: Preliminary results from randomized controlled studies looking into the potential protective role of phytoestrogens on bones suggest that when soy products are consumed in large amounts (40 grams of soy protein and 90 mg of isoflavones daily), they may help to build bone strength and protect against bone loss.

Calcium Essentials

Building bone density and avoiding osteoporosis goes beyond eating dairy products and taking supplements. You can eat a diet full of calcium, but generally your body only absorbs about one-third of what you consume. And absorption declines as we age.

In addition to boosting calcium intake, it's essential to maintain a balanced diet, get certain minerals, and exercise. (See Chapter 5.)

The Color of Health

The phytochemicals (some phytochemicals have antioxidant properties) in whole fruits and vegetables have been shown to help prevent heart disease and cancer. A plant's color is determined by its phytochemicals, which protect the plant and the people who eat it. Vary the colors of vegetables on your plate and you will ensure that you are digesting a healthy variety of these protective phytochemicals.

Orange vegetables, such as carrots and sweet potatoes, contain alpha- and beta-carotene. *Red vegetables* such as tomatoes contain lycopene, while red grapes and blueberries contain anthocyanins. *Dark green vegetables* such as broccoli and kale contain sulforaphane, isothiocyanate, and indoles. Pay particular attention to consuming dark orange and dark green fruits and vegetables, which are loaded with antioxidants.

Although we are still trying to figure out how each of these phytochemicals exerts its protective effects in the body, consuming a variety of them helps to ensure that you will benefit from protection against a variety of toxins.

When eating for bone strength, look for calcium rich foods including dairy products, beans, vegetables, and fruits. Mix and match sources. For instance, soy is a great nondairy alternative (especially if you're lactose intolerant).

The calcium count: Generally, we need more calcium as we age. There are several reasons for this. Because our ability to absorb calcium declines, we need it to help counter bone loss. To assure you're getting enough, keep track of how much calcium you get from your diet. On food labels, calcium content is often given in percentages of daily values (DVs). This is based on a daily recommendation of 1,000 mg. So, if a label says "Calcium 30 percent," that serving has 300 mg of calcium.

To get 1,200 mg of calcium per day, which is the minimum for women if you're age fifty-one or older, you will have to eat or drink three dairy products (about 300–330 mg each) per day (you get 200 mg of calcium from miscellaneous foods). If you are not getting enough calcium in your diet (and even if you are), talk to your clinician about calcium supplements. You don't want to overdose on calcium. But you may need insurance that you're getting and absorbing enough.

Calcium Recommendations

Age	Calcium Intake (range per day)
9–18	1,300–2,500 mg
19–50	1,000–2,500 mg
51 and older	1,200–2,500 mg

Note: The lower number of the recommendations is the minimum, which most people shoot for.

Source: National Institute of Medicine, National Research Council.

Sorting out calcium supplements: Calcium carbonate, calcium citrate malate, or calcium citrate are all good calcium supplements. In general, they are best absorbed when taken with a meal and taken throughout the day in dosages of 500 mg or less.

Calcium carbonate (Tums, Caltrate, Oscal) has the most calcium per pill; therefore you need to take fewer pills, but some people find it constipating. Despite this, calcium carbonate has been found to help alleviate PMS, making it an attractive option. (See Chapter 8.) Calcium citrate malate is the best absorbed by a slight margin but it's more expensive (found in juices or pills). Calcium citrate (Citracal) is well absorbed and does not constipate, but you need many more pills

per day since it has less calcium per pill. If you must take them between meals, calcium citrate is best absorbed.

Calcium absorption: You may not realize it, but vitamin D is essential in
the process of building bone. Vitamin D helps with absorption and
aids in the biochemical transformation of calcium into bone. We get
it from two sources: diet (including supplements) and sun exposure.
The problem is too much sun puts us at risk for skin cancer and few
foods naturally contain significant amounts. The best sources are
saltwater fish and seafood (for example, salmon, tuna, shrimp). Milk,
some cereals, and supplements are often fortified with vitamin D to
prevent deficiency.

After age fifty, our bodies have a tougher time converting this vitamin to its active form, so the daily recommendation is boosted to 400
IU. Magnesium is another important mineral in bone building. It's estimated that you should take half as much magnesium to balance out the
calcium you're taking. For example, if you take 1,000 mg of calcium,
you should take 500 mg of magnesium. Zinc, potassium, vitamin K, vitamin C, manganese, copper, and boron also assist in bone formation.
Check with your clinician to make sure you're getting enough of the es-
sentials either in your diet, in supplement form, or both.

As you work to absorb calcium, watch factors that could be
sabotaging your efforts. Caffeine may increase excretion of calcium.
This is only a factor in those individuals with marginal calcium
intake. Extra sodium in the diet causes calcium excretion. Every
500 mg of sodium over 2,400 mg per day causes the body to excrete
10 mg of calcium. High-phosphorus foods, like carbonated soft
drinks, meat, fish, poultry, and processed cheeses, stop the body from
being able to use the calcium. A study from Boston showed that girls
who drink a lot of soda have weaker and thinner bones compared
with those who drink less. Excess animal protein in the diet causes
the body to excrete calcium. It turns out too much protein can make

the blood acidic, which prompts the body to draw calcium from the bones to neutralize the pH (similar to what Tums does for stomach acid).

Vegans, who eat no animal protein and not many foods high in calcium, were shown not to be at increased risk for osteoporosis in an *American Journal of Clinical Nutrition* study. The no animal protein diet may protect them. The protein effect on bones may also be a reason to reconsider high-protein diets.

Maintaining a Healthy Weight

If you're having a hard time maintaining a healthy weight, the reason is not always unhealthy "junk foods." You can gain weight even while eating healthy foods, by eating large portions. And we often think we're eating the right amount—but it's deceiving!

Portion distortion is an easy trap to fall into. Many serving sizes designated by food manufacturers, even those who produce healthy food, are small and unrealistic for most people. What you consider a serving may be double or triple the size specified on the label. Therefore, determine the number of servings you realistically expect to eat in one sitting, and multiply the calories, grams, and milligrams on the food label by that number. If you're not comfortable measuring your foods refer back to the picture of the plate at the beginning of this chapter. When you fill your plate, try to be sure there is as much low-calorie vegetable as the combined amount of starch and protein. This will help to limit total calories without using measuring utensils.

If you want to lose weight, subtract 250 to 500 calories daily (by eliminating a candy bar or reducing portion size at meals, for example) for a one-half to one-pound weight loss per week. To gain weight, add 250 calories a day. To improve your overall health, follow the guidelines provided in the chart on the next page.

Recommended Nutrient Intake

Nutrient	Recommended Intake
Total calories	Your weight in pounds × 11.4 for weight maintenance
Total fat	25% to 35% of total calories
Saturated fat	12–15 grams/day or less
Other fats	Consume as little trans fats as possible; make sure most of your fat calories come from unsaturated fats
Carbohydrates	50%–60% of total calories (choose whole grain, high fiber sources)
Cholesterol	Keep to less than 300 mg/day
Sodium	Keep to less than 2,000 mg/day
Fiber	Consume 25 grams or more/day
Sugar	Limit sweets to 200 calories/day

Mind Over Matter: Weight Loss

The fact is we equate food with enjoyment and life. So, it makes no sense to treat food as if it were the enemy. Instead improve your relationship with food.

Enjoy in moderation: Although many people worry that desserts are diet-busters, it doesn't have to be that way. To gain one pound of fat, you have to consume 3,500 additional calories. Eating the occasional piece of chocolate cake, at 350 calories, delivers only one-tenth of that amount. (It's habitual intake, day after day, and multiple daily servings that wreak havoc with your weight.) To stay on the safe side, restrict sweet consumption to 200 calories per day or less, about the amount you'd find in one cup of low-fat frozen yogurt or four Fig Newton cookies. Another way to include some treats during a typical week is to use the 80–20 rule: eat healthy foods like fruits, vegetables, whole grains, and fish 80 percent of the time, and the other 20 percent of the time enjoy foods that you don't regularly have.

Set realistic goals: If you're thinking about losing weight, choose a goal that is realistic and achievable. A reasonable goal is to try to reduce your weight by 10 percent over six months, and then maintain the new weight before attempting to lose any more. (So if you weigh 180 pounds, losing 18 pounds is reasonable.) Also, don't weigh yourself more than once a week. This will help you to avoid the emotional roller coaster of watching your weight go up and down. Also, don't use your weight as the only marker for success. Actually, lost inches are a better marker for body fat loss. So notice how your bra and pants feel as additional feedback to your progress. (See Chapter 5 for tips on accurate measurements.)

Plan for a slow burn: People who crash diet and initially lose a large amount of weight are losing mostly fluid and muscle tissue, and tend to gain weight back very quickly. To prevent your resting metabolism from dropping as you diet, eat at regular intervals throughout the day but reduce portions and calories.

Keep moving: People who are able to lose weight and keep it off are those who exercise regularly. Choose something that you enjoy and will fit into your normal routine. A mix of aerobic and anaerobic is best for long-term weight management.

Mind/body approaches to watching your waistline

When you find yourself reaching for food when you don't really need it, try this four-step strategy: Stop, Breathe, Reflect, and Choose.

1. *Stop.* Stop yourself before automatically eating food.
2. *Breathe.* Do a mini! This will not only relax you but will prevent you from automatically eating.
3. *Reflect.* Why do you want to eat at this moment? Is it hunger or because you feel depressed, anxious, stressed, or bored?
4. *Choose.* If you are eating because of a negative emotion, not hunger, try to choose a non-food-related activity to make yourself feel better (for example, take a walk, practice the relaxation response, or call a friend).

This strategy helps to reduce impulse eating because it gives you time to think and make a different choice.

Another useful strategy is using sticker reminders. Place stickers (we use blue dots) in strategic places where you keep food or where you regularly eat (on your refrigerator, on the back of the cookie cupboard door, etc.). The sticker is a cue to you to stop, breathe, and reflect why you want to eat that food before automatically reaching in and grabbing it. You'll be the only one who knows what this sticker means. If you think about why you reach for a particular food, you may stop yourself if you realize that you want to eat because of negative emotions rather than hunger. If you don't stop to think about it, then you'll eat that food 100 percent of the time. The stickers can help you reduce mindless or emotional eating.

If you truly are hungry, choose a healthy snack or a small portion of a high-calorie food and eat it mindfully.

If you do catch yourself before emotionally eating you can try a non-food activity to improve your mood. Identify some so that you can use them the next time you feel bad and want to eat.

Identifying hidden calories

Sometimes calories are tucked away. We think we're eating healthy at a buffet, but we're not. Here are some common, but often unconsidered, calorie sources:

Don't be fooled by "fat free": Don't think you can eat larger portions of low-fat desserts, because these are often loaded with sugar and have as many calories per serving as high-fat desserts. (The same is true for items like baked tortilla chips, which have about the same calories per chip as fried tortilla chips.) Eat too many of these "low-fat" alternatives, and you'll consume extra calories that are converted into— you guessed it—body fat. To limit portions of items like ice cream, use cones (which hold less than a bowl) or teacups. You can also choose fruit instead of cookies or pastry, and obtain an added bonus in the form of fiber, nutrients, and phytochemicals.

Beware of hidden fats: Choose a mixed green salad for lunch, and then drown it in salad dressing, and you may end up ingesting more calories than if you had a hamburger. Hidden fats are everywhere: in

More Good Protein Is Not Better

Although fish and poultry contain fewer calories and saturated fat per ounce than red meat that doesn't mean you can eat larger portion sizes. Portions of any type of meat should be about three to four-and-a-half ounces, the size of one to one and one-half decks of playing cards. To understand how eating large portions of healthy protein may affect weight loss, consider these two scenarios.

Hamburger	Haddock
3 ounces	6 ounces
90 calories/ounce	55 calories/ounce
Calories consumed: 270	Calories consumed: 330

For weight loss, it would be better to eat a small hamburger than a large piece of haddock. These calculations were done using a low-fat fish. If you substituted a fatty fish, the calories go up even higher (closer to 500 calories for a six-ounce piece of salmon).

baked goods, in condiments like sour cream, cream cheese, salad dressing, and mayonnaise. They can also lurk in seemingly healthy choices in restaurants, such as Caesar salads and tunafish salad sandwiches (often the selections highest in calories are smothered in dressing and mayonnaise). Choose light or low-fat condiments, dressings, and sauces.

Liquid calories: Drink just one can of sugar-laden soda a day, without decreasing calories or increasing activity, and you could gain fifteen pounds by the end of the year. Several studies even suggest that drinking high-calorie beverages may actually prompt you to consume more food at a meal. Water is always the best choice; 36–48 fl. oz. per day is recommended.

A regular beer has 150 calories, four ounces of dry wine has 80 calories, and a two-and-a-half-ounce martini has 156 calories. Eliminate one beer each day for a full year, and you could lose fifteen pounds by the end of the year without doing anything else. To cut down on calories, choose sugar-free soft drinks, and light beer instead of regular beer. If you prefer wine, try a wine spritzer, which is half wine, half seltzer water, and cuts the calories in half. When out socially, try alternating alcoholic with low-calorie nonalcoholic beverages.

The Benefits of Alcohol?

For women over age fifty, there is some confusion over the benefits of alcohol. In various studies, one drink a day of beer or wine reduces your risk for heart disease. On the other hand, more than one drink a day can also increase your risk for breast cancer and risk for fracture due to falls. As always, check with your clinician.

Eat Mindfully to Eat Well

Can you remember whether or not you enjoyed your last meal? How long did it take you to eat the meal? Did you realize if you were full or not? What are some adjectives to describe the food in your mouth as you ate it? The answers to these questions indicate whether you are a mindless eater or a mindful eater.

Americans often eat while doing other things. In this era of multitasking, one thing that gets shoved aside is mealtime. Lunch becomes just another annoyance that takes time away from more important tasks, rather than being viewed as a welcome and enjoyable break.

It doesn't have to be that way. If you set aside time to eat, without being distracted by other activities, you will find that you eat less but enjoy it more.

To become a mindful eater, separate eating from your other activities. Create a nice setting and try to take at least twenty minutes to eat. This allows you to savor and appreciate the flavor and texture of food in your mouth and it gives your stomach time to fill sufficiently and send chemical signals to your brain indicating that you are satiated. In the end, there are many benefits:

1. You will eat less food.
2. You will become more aware of feeling satisfied and avoid negative feelings caused by overeating and indigestion.
3. You will be able to indulge in an occasional moderate portion of a high-calorie food.
4. Your digestion will improve, since the food is chewed more thoroughly.
5. You will taste and enjoy what you eat.

Want to make a meal mindful? Try this: Eat a meal or snack as slowly as possible. Pay attention to the tastes and textures that you are experiencing. Savor the food(s) so that you really appreciate the flavors and experience the enjoyment of eating. Now take a moment to think what you noticed. How did the food taste? (Sweet? Salty? Tart?) How did it feel on your tongue? (Coarse? Smooth? A little of both?) Did you chew slowly so you could savor the food before swallowing? Did you enjoy the aroma before putting the food in your mouth? How long did it take you to eat the food?

One of our most popular and tastiest exercises practices mindfulness using a chocolate kiss. It's truly amazing how much pleasure and enjoyment you can get out of just a few calories! When eating mindfully, you get more from your food, more enjoyment from eating, and you usually end up eating less.

We encourage women to think of food as a friend, not an enemy. The right foods, in the right balance, can make you feel better and live longer—one of the best prescriptions going!

CHAPTER 7

Postmenopausal Hormone Therapy

If you picked up this book, you are likely looking for alternatives to hormones for managing menopause. Or you may simply want to know all of your options. In either case, it's good to understand the medical approach to hormone therapy and how studies over the years have shed light on its effects. Mention the topic and two words come to mind: confusion and controversy. It is controversial because recent studies show that use of hormone therapy is associated with an increased risk of breast cancer and heart attack. It is confusing because hormone therapy is still very much a part of the medical picture and there are many formulas to choose from. How do you sort it all out? Today, hormones have become part of a balancing act.

Meagan had trouble getting through her day due to severe hot flashes. For her, short-term hormone therapy has allowed her to manage her symptoms. Crystal, on the other hand, is strongly opposed to taking hormones—even temporarily—because of a fear of breast cancer. Dorine has opted for a low-dose vaginal tablet, which offers relief from vaginal dryness without some of the risks associated with systemic hormone therapy. All three women have made decisions based on what's right for them.

As with all medications, women and their clinicians need to decide whether the benefits outweigh the risks. A woman's age, symptoms, menopausal status, risk factors, and family history weigh into the decision that is right for her alone. In a mind/body approach, we advise women to make a commitment to a healthy lifestyle and, depending on the severity of their symptoms, make informed decisions about any medications they take. The goal of this chapter is to help you navigate the changing hormonal landscape and make sense of medical studies, so that you can make informed decisions about your own health.

In some situations estrogen can improve hot flashes and vaginal dryness, and in some situations may improve sleep and mood. There may also be selected indications for its long-term use (see Chapter 2). While we emphasize lifestyle approaches in mind/body medicine, we recognize the importance of medication when needed. After all, maximizing our quality of life is essential to our well-being. There has never been much doubt that estrogen relieves certain symptoms. But medical opinion has swayed back and forth between recommending and discouraging its long-term use. Thus, it's been a roller coaster ride for women taking (or thinking about) hormone therapy (HT). As of this writing, the weight of the evidence is against long-term use of postmenopausal hormone therapy for prevention of chronic conditions because of an increased risk for both breast cancer and heart attack. The latest consensus follows decades of changing opinions.

On the way up, estrogen was popularized in the 1960s and 1970s as a treatment for menopausal symptoms and even a "cure" for menopause, as described in Dr. Robert A. Wilson's 1966 book, *Feminine Forever*. Estrogen was promoted by some doctors as a risk-free way to remain young. Then came the first cold dash of reality. In 1975, studies linked estrogen to an increased risk of uterine cancer. However, it was then shown that this risk was eliminated when estrogen was combined with progestin. Thus, advocates of estrogen replacement therapy became advocates of combined estrogen and progestin therapy, which we discuss in more detail later in this chapter.

In the 1980s, hormone therapy again gained momentum when research suggested combined estrogen and progestin therapy could help prevent chronic diseases including heart disease, osteoporosis, and colon cancer. By the mid-1990s, most published evidence favored the long-term use of combined hormone therapy. At the time, physicians found the heart protective benefits of estrogen compelling. At the same time, there has always been concern about hormone therapy and breast cancer risk because estrogen can promote some forms of the disease. Heart disease is the number one killer of women, killing six times more women than breast cancer. It would make good sense to prescribe something that would reduce that risk. Add in the benefits of preventing osteoporosis and colon cancer and it appeared that the benefits of staying on hormone therapy exceeded the risks well past the age of menopause. Yet, the story, as most women know, did not end there.

A dramatic turn of events came in the summer of 2002 with the release of results from the Women's Health Initiative—the largest clinical trial ever performed relative to menopause and midlife health. The results showed that not only could hormone therapy increase a woman's risk of breast cancer, but it also increased her risk for heart attack, stroke, blood clots, and probable dementia. The stunning news quickly dismantled the idea that hormone therapy was a "cure-all."

Today hormones are no longer viewed as a "magic" pill. Weighing the decision is a personal choice.

The Benefits and Risks of Hormone Therapy (HT)

The Women's Health Initiative showed that the most commonly prescribed combination of estrogen and progestin (Prempro) has definite bone benefits and it reduces the risk of colon cancer. However, it also carries an increased risk of breast cancer, heart attacks, strokes, and blood clots, and possibly dementia. The news was dramatic because earlier studies had shown hormone therapy (HT) to be heart protective and millions of women had been taking HT, at least in part, for the prevention of heart disease.

When Nora learned that she had slight bone loss and her doctor realized there was heart disease in her family, her doctor advised her to consider HT. Based on the scientific evidence at the time, it seemed the perfect way to reduce her risk of heart attack and at the same time protect her bones. Three years later, she was diagnosed with stage one breast cancer. It was invasive but treatable. Judy, on the other hand, had suffered a heart attack. Since then, she had been taking hormones hoping to prevent a second one. In ten years she had experienced no problems, but she quickly discontinued hormone therapy after the Women's Health Initiative study was released.

Why do earlier findings conflict with newer data? One of the reasons for the turnabout is the type of studies upon which these conclusions have been based. As we describe some of the key studies conducted over the years, you'll see why opinions about hormones have changed.

The Nurses' Health Study

Some of the strongest early evidence in support of long-term postmenopausal HT came from the Nurses' Health Study—a broad study that has followed 120,000 nurses over more than twenty-five years. As you consider this early data it is important to keep in mind that the

Nurses' Health Study is an observational study. Observational studies do just that, observe. This form of research has played a major role in our understanding of health issues. But it does have limitations and inherent flaws.

In the mid 1980s, researchers in the Nurses' Health Study first reported that women on estrogen therapy were less likely to experience serious heart disease when compared with women who did not take hormones. Their conclusions held up even when the investigators accounted for other risk factors including smoking, being overweight, and a family history of heart disease. Through the 1990s, this study continued to report similar results, including data suggesting that adding progestin didn't affect the apparently compelling cardiovascular benefits of postmenopausal hormones. The Nurses' Health Study also found that while women were taking HT, they were about 35 percent less likely to develop colon cancer than women who had never taken the hormones. They also reduced their risk of osteoporosis-related fractures.

However, in 1990, the Nurses' Health Study reported that women who use estrogen face an increased risk of breast cancer. Several subsequent reports from the Nurses' Health Study and other large and respected observational studies found the same thing. Many of the same studies that showed an increased risk of breast cancer from HT, however, also continued to show that combined estrogen and progestin therapy protected women against osteoporosis, colon cancer, and heart disease.

Another potential risk found during the Nurses' Health Study was that estrogen, with or without progestin, increased the likelihood of having the gallbladder removed. Estrogen's ability to raise the level of cholesterol in bile produced by the liver and stored in the gallbladder promotes the growth of gallstones. The higher the dose of hormone therapy and the longer its use, the more likely a woman was to have the surgery. Five years after they stopped, women who had used hormones still had a higher risk of gallbladder removal than women who never had taken hormones. At the time, observational studies suggested that the benefits of HT might outweigh the risks. This conclusion was, in large part, based on the assumption that HT reduced the risk of heart attack.

The Heart and Estrogen/Progestin Replacement Study

In 1999, an alarming study was published. The Heart and Estrogen/Progestin Replacement Study (HERS) gave combined hormone therapy or a placebo (inactive or "fake" medication) at random to postmenopausal women with known heart disease. This is known as a secondary prevention study. HERS, designed to *prevent* further heart disease in women *who already had it,* did not show the protective effect of combined hormone therapy that previous studies had indicated. Indeed, it showed that new heart problems occurred more often in the first two years of treatment, compared with women assigned to take the placebo.

Many doctors initially interpreted the HERS study as showing two things. First, combined hormone therapy might increase the risk

Understanding Observational Studies

In observational studies such as the Nurses' Health Study, a large group of people is studied for many years. Information is carefully collected about their lifestyles, medications, and other factors. Any diseases that subsequently develop are noted. The drawback of observational studies is that the participants who choose to take a particular medicine (in this case, hormones) may be different in important ways from the people who opt not to take the medicine. For example, they might be more health conscious to start with, and/or have healthier lifestyles. It could be these factors, and not the use of hormones, that are responsible for the differences in outcome of these two groups.

Randomized Controlled Trials

Randomized controlled trials are considered the gold standard of scientific methods used to determine the impact of medication or other types of medical treatment.

Participants are purposely diversified, selected, and randomly assigned medications or placebos. This provides a more accurate way of gathering pertinent data than other studies. Because participants don't know what they're taking, it lessens the chances of bias. In addition, purposely diversifying and randomizing participants helps to ensure that other factors that can affect data (example: one group exercises more than another) are limited.

of new heart problems in women who *already had heart disease.* Second, combined therapy might increase the risk of heart problems in any postmenopausal woman for the first two years of taking it, although thereafter it might have a protective effect. Thus, many doctors continued to advise postmenopausal women without known heart disease to continue on treatment.

HERS raises an important point when understanding medical studies. Is a medication being taken to control (or avoid the worsening of) a preexisting condition? This is called *secondary prevention—* for example, when a person who has had a heart attack starts taking a cholesterol-lowering drug, along with a beta-blocker to prevent a second attack. Or is it intended to prevent the initial occurrence in an otherwise healthy woman? This is called *primary prevention—*for example, when a woman without known heart disease takes a cholesterol-lowering drug to lower her risk of cardiovascular problems.

The Women's Health Initiative

The Women's Health Initiative—a randomized clinical trial—comprises multiple "arms" (specific studies) and has enrolled more than

161,000 women ages fifty through seventy-nine. One of these studies evaluated the risks and benefits of combined hormone therapy with estrogen and progestin in *preventing* long-term chronic diseases in apparently healthy women (primary prevention study). Researchers assigned 16,608 women to either Prempro (a particular formulation of estrogen and progestin) or placebo.

Interestingly, much of the data from the Women's Health Initiative supported conclusions drawn from earlier observational studies. Hormone therapy slightly increased breast cancer risk, lowered the risk of osteoporosis and related hip fractures, and reduced the chances of developing colon cancer. But on two issues it came to an opposite conclusion from most observational studies on hormones. First, postmenopausal hormone therapy in the form known as Prempro was likely to *increase*, not decrease, the risk of heart disease. Secondly, it was likely to *increase,* not decrease, the risk of probable dementia. The rates of heart disease, breast cancer, stroke and pulmonary embolism (blood clots in the lung) were not high, but they were increased.

Why would physicians and women take particular notice of the Women's Health Initiative data? Because of the study's design. The Women's Health Initiative is a randomized controlled clinical trial, which is considered the gold standard of scientific methods used to determine the impact of medication or other types of medical treatment. These differ from observational studies in that the *study design* (not the participants) randomly assigns a particular treatment to some of the participants and a placebo to the others. Typically neither the participants nor their doctors nor the people running the study know which participants took the medicine (in this case, hormones) and which were taking placebo until the study is over. Most clinicians take the results of a randomized trial over those of observational studies when results are different. No one is sure why the Women's Health Initiative results regarding heart disease were so different from the results of many observational studies. Most people assume the answer rests with the superiority of randomized trials in uncovering the truth. However, the participants in the Women's Health Initiative tended to be older—and initiated HT later in life—than the women who participated in the earlier observational studies. And there may prove to be other differences between studies as well.

As a result of the conclusions of the Women's Health Initiative investigators, doctors no longer recommend—and many women no longer accept—hormone therapy as a preventive treatment for later life's ills. It is important to note, this research was not intended to assess hormone therapy's effects on symptoms or quality of life in women with severe menopausal symptoms.

Levels of Evidence

Needless to say, the more rigorous and solid a study, the more weight it carries. Thousands of studies are underway at any given time. Some of these are very small and limited in their ability to control what is being studied. When you read "Studies show . . ." find out what *kind* of studies, before you use the information to make a decision regarding your health.

Considering "levels of evidence" is like reviewing a report card. Scientific studies can be "graded" based on the scientific rigor of the study design. So how do they stack up?

- The highest level of evidence is a *randomized controlled trial,* such as the Women's Health Initiative.
- The next level of evidence includes *observational studies* and *controlled trials without randomization.*
- The lowest level of evidence is *opinions of experts* and studies that describe the experience of a few patients *(anecdotal evidence).* The effect of a medicine or treatment on one person can't be generalized to everyone.

How risky is postmenopausal hormone therapy?

When the Women's Health Initiative study (WHI) says hormone therapy raises the risk of breast cancer by 26 percent and heart attack by 29 percent that sounds like a lot. But what does that mean for you?

Medical studies typically report two kinds of risk: relative risk and absolute risk. Often, news about recently published research focuses on relative risk—and doesn't tell you about absolute risk. You need to know both numbers in order to make a judgment about the level of risk you're willing to accept.

Relative risk is the percentage change in risk (increase or decrease) in one group of people taking a particular drug (or having a particular treatment) compared to a group that doesn't take the drug or treatment. To understand relative risk, think about this. Let's say one in a million people get a disease. Sounds like a very slim chance? You're right. But if the number becomes 1.5 in a million, there has been a 50 percent increase, boosting relative risk to 50 percent. *Absolute risk* is the actual number of individuals who develop a specific disease during a specified time period—let's use the same 1.5 in a million. So, even though your relative risk has risen significantly, your absolute risk has only risen by 0.5, meaning you still have a 999,998.5 chance of *not* getting the disease.

To better clarify absolute risk, we use real life data from the Women's Health Initiative. In the WHI data, the absolute risk over one year was 8 more breast cancers among 10,000 women who take hormone therapy versus those who don't. In other words, for every 10,000 women taking estrogen plus progestin pills, 38 developed breast cancer each year compared to 30 breast cancers for every 10,000 women taking placebo pills each year. So, despite the fact that there was a 26 percent increase in relative risk, it is still a small absolute risk.

Some people find it helpful to "visualize" absolute risk. For example, imagine a sports arena with 10,000 seats filled with women watching a tennis match. Now, imagine that eight of those women will develop breast cancer, and you might be one of those eight. Does that feel like a high risk or a low risk? Different people will probably give different answers. However you might answer, you really need to know both the relative and absolute risks to determine the right answer for you.

The Absolute and Relative Risks of Combined Estrogen and Progestin (Prempro) as Reported by the Women's Health Initiative

Number of patients who will become ill out of 10,000 taking Prempro

Incidents of Illness	Placebo	HT	Absolute Risk of HT	Relative Risk of HT
Breast cancer	30	38	8 more	26% increase
Heart attack	30	37	7 more	29% increase
Stroke	21	29	8 more	41% increase
Blood clots	16	34	18 more	50% increase
Colon cancer	16	10	6 fewer	37% less
Hip fracture	15	10	5 fewer	34% less

Note: Results are averaged using 10,000 women in order to register risks in whole integers. The results are based on actual incidents that would occur over a one-year time span.

Source: Adapted from The Women's Health Initiative, National Institutes of Health. For updates: http://www.whi.org

Time is also a consideration. Again, using the WHI trial as an example: over the 5.2 years of the trial, the cumulative number of adverse events in women taking the hormone combination was 100 per

10,000 (1 in 100 women). This is still a small risk, but it shows that risks can add up over time. In the case of breast cancer, there was no increased risk until four years into the study. For heart disease, the opposite was true. Most adverse heart related events happened within one to two years, then began to taper.

It is important to stress that the findings may not apply to women who have had hysterectomies and are taking only estrogen. In addition, it is unknown to what extent the WHI findings apply to women taking hormone products other than Prempro; however, the FDA has advised that all estrogen and progestin products be considered to have similar risks until proven otherwise. Studies evaluating estrogen alone, including the estrogen-only trial of the Women's Health Initiative, as well as other hormone combinations, continue.*

Making a Decision about Hormone Therapy

Whether you've taken hormones for fifteen years or are thinking about taking them short-term to help hot flashes, the days of "take this pill and call me in the morning" are and should be in the past. Women still take hormones, but today most of them carefully weigh the risks and benefits with their doctors. There are literally hundreds of hormone preparations and today they can be tailored to meet each woman's needs. The best approach: be informed.

Current evidence argues against long-term hormone therapy to reduce the risk of cardiovascular disease, osteoporosis, and dementia in most women. But short-term HT can help women deal with menopausal symptoms. Data from future studies may change this—it is possible that some women would benefit from long-term HT, while others would be subjected to unusual risks from even short-term HT.

* Results from the estrogen-only trial of the Women's Health Initiative are expected in 2005.

So what should you do? Work with your clinician to evaluate your menopausal symptoms, your risk for bone loss, breast cancer, and heart disease, and your preference for a treatment regimen. How do you feel about taking hormones? If the risk of breast cancer is one of the most important considerations for you in deciding whether to take hormone therapy your clinician can help you calculate your risk. Together, you will have to weigh a number of factors in your risk profile—for example, a family history of breast cancer, whether you started menstruating early, and whether you've had children—with the severity of your symptoms to arrive at an informed decision. So far, doctors don't fully understand the degree to which the increased risk from combined hormone therapy interacts with a woman's other risk factors.

Here are some general guidelines from the Women's Health Initiative to consider as well:

- If menopausal symptoms adversely affect your quality of life, you might want to consider HT. The Women's Health Initiative was not designed to specifically examine women with severe menopausal symptoms. Thus, no conclusions have been drawn. However, it has been specifically stated that the short-term use of HT for symptoms is an area where the benefits may outweigh the risks for an individual woman.
- Don't take HT for the purpose of preventing cardiovascular disease.
- For osteoporosis prevention, talk to your doctor. You may want to consider alternative medications.

Please note that the 2002 Women's Health Initiative data do not apply to you if you have had a hysterectomy and are taking estrogen without a progestin, or if you have early menopause. If either applies to you, talk to your clinician about the potential risks and benefits of HT.

Taking Hormone Therapy

The goal of hormone therapy is to treat symptoms using the lowest dose that is effective, for the shortest time possible. The amount and type of hormone is specifically formulated according to the symptom. There are different preparations, different routes of administration, and variability in response from woman to woman. Formulas range from local preparations for the relief of vaginal dryness to pills or patches for the relief of hot flashes. The lowest dose of oral estrogen so far shown to reduce hot flashes is 0.3 mg of conjugated estrogens. This level has also been shown to protect against bone loss in most women. For hot flashes, women usually feel some relief within the first month, but it can take several months to feel complete relief, and there may be some side effects, including vaginal bleeding (if you still have a uterus), nausea, breast tenderness, headache, mood swings, and changes in libido. Because there are a variety of prescription products and doses to choose from, you may need to try different products at different doses and regimens until you find the best choice for your symptoms and health concerns.

Most women in the United States take estrogen in pill form, but it's also available in patches and vaginal creams, rings, and tablets. While different forms of delivery alter the dosage levels, there is no evidence that any particular FDA approved form of hormone therapy is in any way superior. Generally speaking, equivalent doses of estrogen are believed to have equivalent effects.

FDA-Approved Postmenopausal Hormone Options

Type of Hormone	Brand Name
Estrogen Pills	
Conjugated equine estrogens	Premarin
Synthetic conjugated estrogens	Cenestin

Estrogen Pills (*continued*)

Esterified estrogens	Estratab
	Menest
Estradiol	Estrace
	Various generics
Estropipate	Ortho-Est
	Ogen
	Various generics
Ethinyl estradiol	Estinyl

Estrogen Skin Patches, Gels, and Creams

Estradiol matrix patch	Alora
	Climara
	Esclim
	Vivelle
	Vivelle-Dot
Estradiol reservoir patch	Estraderm
Estradiol topical emulsion	Estrasorb

Estrogen Used Vaginally

Creams

Estradiol	Estrace Vaginal Cream
Conjugated equine estrogens	Premarin Vaginal Cream

Ring

Estradiol	Estring
	FemRing (full dose therapy for hot flashes as well as vaginal symptoms)

Tablet

Estradiol	Vagifem

Type of Hormone	Brand Name
Progestogens	
Progestins: Oral	
Medroxyprogesterone	Amen
acetate (MPA)	Curretab
	Cycrin
	Provera
	Various generics
Norethindrone	Micronor
	Nor-QD
Norethindrone acetate	Aygestin
	Norlutate
	Generic
Norgestrel	Ovrette
Micronized progesterone USP	Prometrium
(in peanut oil)	
Progestins: Local	
Levonorgestrel/IUD	Mirena
Progesterone vaginal gel	Crinone

Combination Estrogen-Progestogen Products	
Oral	
Conjugated equine estrogens +	Premphase
medroxyprogesterone acetate	Prempro
	Low-dose Prempro
Ethinyl estradiol + norethindrone	Femhrt
acetate	
Estradiol + norethindrone acetate	Activella
Estradiol + norgestimate	Ortho-Prefest
Skin patches	
Estradiol + norethindrone acetate	CombiPatch

Taking only estrogen is referred to as *unopposed estrogen therapy*. Doctors prescribe it only for women who have had a hysterectomy because unopposed estrogen greatly increases the risk of cancer of the uterine lining (endometrial cancer). As mentioned earlier, *combined therapy* adds a form of progesterone to estrogen. Progesterone can be taken in synthetic form (called progestin) or in "natural" form. Adding a progestin to estrogen therapy reduces the risk of developing uterine cancer to the same level as someone not taking hormones.

Some women cannot tolerate the adverse effects of progestin—bloating, moodiness and irritability, and sometimes spotty menstrual bleeding—and may stop taking the progestin and continue taking the estrogen only. This is a dangerous practice for a woman who still has a uterus. The two most common approaches for taking estrogen and a progestin are *cyclical* and *continuous* therapy. Cyclic therapy involves taking progestin for part of the cycle and can result in withdrawal bleeding. Continuous combined therapy uses a constant dose of estrogen and progestin that you take every day. Over a period of time, continuous combined therapy can result in no bleeding.

Hormone patches: While pills are the most common way to take HT, transdermal patches can also deliver standard dosages of estrogen through the skin and into the bloodstream. Patches are worn discreetly on the abdomen or buttocks. Reservoir patches have a waterproof backing and a small supply of the drug that's suspended in alcohol. The alcohol carries the drug through a membrane in the patch and into the skin. Matrix patches deliver estrogen through a layer of gel. This type of patch is thinner and less bulky than reservoir patches.

Most of the estrogen-only patches marketed in the United States deliver estradiol. Estradiol enters the bloodstream rapidly, quickly reaching target tissues. As a result, doses can be lower than those used in oral estrogen. Another reason the patch contains lower doses is because the hormone isn't broken down by digestion, as it is when you swallow it in a pill.

Because estrogen delivered via a patch bypasses the digestive system, it may not improve the cholesterol profile to the same extent as pills. But it may be less likely to cause gallstones. Women with sensitive skin may find patches cause irritation. Women with an intact uterus should use a form of progesterone in addition to the estrogen patch. A patch that contains estrogen and progestin (CombiPatch) is available. Usually each patch is effective for three to seven days. Patches are usually more expensive than pills, but there is one generic estrogen patch available.

Vaginal forms of hormone therapy: One way to relieve symptoms of vaginal dryness and irritation is to use local preparations: creams, rings, tablets. (See Chapter 8.) These products treat only the local tissues of the vagina and typically do not treat systemic symptoms such as hot flashes. You don't absorb nearly as much hormone from these as you do from pills or patches, so they do not carry the same benefits and risks as estrogen taken by pill or patch. Only small doses are needed to relieve vaginal dryness. Even though these estrogen products are used in low doses in the vagina, they can still stimulate precancerous changes in the uterus. For this reason, they may need to be opposed with progestin unless a woman has had her uterus removed. Estrogen cream should not be used as a lubricant before intercourse because it can be absorbed through a partner's skin.

Birth control pills

Despite erratic ovulation and a decline in fertility, it is still possible to get pregnant during perimenopause. Clinicians may prescribe birth control pills for perimenopausal women because they are an effective contraceptive method and have noncontraceptive benefits as well. Birth control pills suppress ovarian function and prevent ovulation. As a result, they can smooth out the hormonal swings characteristic of this time. This can also help manage irregular bleeding and painful periods, and reduce hot flashes.

Research shows that the estrogen in birth control pills also slows the rate of bone loss. Longer use appears to help reduce the risk for endometrial and ovarian cancers when used by premenopausal women. However, it takes two years of use to gain protection against endometrial cancer, and three years of use to gain protection against ovarian cancer. Women who use birth control pills short-term to help alleviate menopausal symptoms may not get these protective benefits.

The FDA has not approved birth control pills specifically for the treatment of menopausal symptoms; however, decades of good clinical experience have led many clinicians to prescribe them for this purpose. While there are no solid data indicating which women may benefit from birth control pills, there are some women who should not take them. Women should not take birth control pills if they:

- are over age 35 and smoke
- have high blood pressure
- have a history of blood clots or stroke
- have cancers that may be stimulated by estrogen or progesterone
- have unexplained vaginal bleeding
- could be pregnant

Some women take birth control pills consistently through their mid- to late forties for contraceptive purposes. In this case, a woman might *not* experience (or not noticeably experience) the symptoms that signal the menopausal transition. For example, because birth control pills help regulate menstruation, one of the first signs of menopause—irregular periods—is obscured, although some women may notice hot flashes or worsening headaches during the placebo week (the week the inactive pills are taken).

Birth control pills contain the same hormones as HT, but at much higher doses. Because the risks associated with these hormones—cardiovascular risks in particular—increase with age, it isn't wise to stay on them indefinitely. If you've been on the pills long-term for contraceptive purposes or if your clinician has prescribed them for you to help manage perimenopausal symptoms, how do you know when to stop taking them? This presents a bit of a conundrum. Because FSH levels (see Chapter 2) can stay suppressed for as long as six weeks after the last birth control pill has been taken, this test isn't very practical. Menstrual history isn't a good guide either, because the pill masks the irregular bleeding so typical of the perimenopause. Because by age fifty-five only 2 percent of women have *not* gone through the transition, some clinicians feel comfortable having healthy, nonsmoking women who are at low risk for ill effects from birth control pills stay on them until their early to mid-fifties—when the probability of menopause is high. If you're in your late forties or early fifties and have been on birth control pills, talk with your clinician about how long you should continue—and how to best determine whether you're approaching menopause.

"Natural" hormone therapy

Many women are intrigued by the idea of "natural" hormone therapy. As we've learned more about the potential risks of "standard" postmenopausal hormone therapy, women are looking for alternatives. And many instinctively believe that "natural" is good and "synthetic" is bad. This is where it gets confusing. What is "natural" and what is "synthetic"? We often consider "natural" as that derived from animal, plant, or mineral sources instead of being created in a laboratory. Using this definition, many hormones could be considered natural. For instance, many standard HT formulations are derived from the urine of pregnant mares. Yet they aren't usually referred to as "natural." Similarly, the phytoestrogens in soy appear to have estrogenic effects. Food is natural, but eating soy is not usually considered a part of natural hormone therapy.

So what are natural hormones? Typically the term refers to a variety of hormonal preparations that are derived from plants like soybeans and wild yams. Most have undergone some chemical processing and are formulated to mimic a variety of hormones including estrogen (estradiol, estriol, and estrone), progesterone, and testosterone. Most natural hormones are *bio-identical* to human hormones, which means they have the same molecular or biochemical structure as a woman's own natural hormones. Many women and clinicians believe bio-identical hormones have fewer side effects than synthetics. Unfortunately, most have not undergone rigorous study. Some have gone through the FDA approval process (for example, Prometrium and Estrace), but most have not. "Natural" hormones may have some of the same safety issues as "standard" hormone therapy. Some combinations may contain significant amounts of estrogen, requiring the use of progesterone to protect against endometrial cancer. There may be other risks as well. Advocates suggest that natural hormones are significantly safer and do not increase the risk of breast and endometrial cancers. However, there is no current evidence to support these claims.

Like standard hormone therapy, natural hormone therapy may be prescribed. Since the formulations are not usually FDA-approved, and require some preparation, a *compounding* pharmacy is typically involved. At a compounding pharmacy, pharmacists prepare the hormones (on-site) into various routes of administration, including capsules, tablets, creams, or an injectable form.

While many women like using compounded products to tailor their treatment, if you're considering this form of treatment, you should be aware of a few things. First, although some clinicians prescribe these products by testing a woman's hormone levels periodically, this is of limited use because no one knows exactly what hormone level to aim for, and hormone levels fluctuate. Second, it should also be noted that there is very little data on the safety or effectiveness of compounded hormonal preparations. Because they are largely unregulated, the contents and absorption rates of these hormones can vary in some cases, making it difficult to know exactly what you're getting.

When reviewing your options, note that many types of FDA-approved bio-identical hormone therapies are available. For estrogens, the possibilities include oral, transdermal (patch), and vaginal preparations. For progestins, they include the natural progesterone product Prometrium. If you're interested in "natural" hormone therapy, talk with your clinician. Ask about the latest research on these preparations and whether he or she has experience prescribing natural hormones or advising patients about their use.

Stopping Hormone Therapy

If you've been taking hormone therapy and feel ready to discontinue it for any reason, talk with your doctor. There's really no "standard" guideline for stopping hormone therapy. Some women simply stop without noticeable difficulty. For others, going "cold turkey" may lead to a recurrence of some menopausal symptoms, especially hot flashes, which may return with a vengeance. If a form of progesterone is part of your regimen, it's important to continue taking it as long as you take estrogen. To avoid complications and lessen problems with discontinuation, it's best to work with your doctor.

Staying Informed

As the information on hormones is continually being updated, it's best to stay educated about your options. New hormone therapies are in the works and studies continue to review effectiveness and safety issues. In Chapter 8, "Managing Symptoms," we take a closer look at how specific hormone therapies might fit into an integrated mind/body approach to dealing with menopause. If you are opposed to taking hormones, you will find there are many lifestyle and nonhormonal options. Our advice: read on, try lifestyle approaches, and decide what works for you.

CHAPTER 8

Managing Symptoms

For Jackie, the time had arrived. A hot flash was rolling in that would leave her reaching for napkins. "I would break out in a perspiring sweat. I'd have to mop my face. I'd be totally soaked," she recalled. "At night I would wake up drenched and would have to change."

Meanwhile, Sherry experiences her hot flashes differently. "I call them warms." "The heat goes up my back. I may have to take a sweater off, but they're nothing that extreme." Sherry has no negative emotions about menopause.

In the sometimes unfair and confusing realm of fluctuating hormones, it seems menopause is not an equal opportunity transition. The range of experience is immense. Most women tolerate a variety of symptoms with few problems and without medication. If you turned immediately to this chapter, you may not be among those. The good news is that the options for handling menopausal symptoms are growing. The challenge is deciding what's right for you.

Mind/body medicine focuses on our personal strengths, behavior, and intuition as part of a comprehensive approach to manage symptoms. In the context of menopause, this involves knowing your body, your options, and your values. Are your hot flashes mildly annoying or the cause of great distress? Would you want to take medication? How do you feel about making lifestyle changes? Are you confused about what works and what doesn't?

We have found the answer does not lie in one product or prescription. New medications may offer great help to many women, but they are not the sole solution. There are a variety of ways to deal with the complex interactions among perimenopausal symptoms. An integrated approach includes lifestyle changes along with prescription and nonprescription therapies.

Mind/body medicine is based on scientific evidence. That means the methods and therapies we recognize as effective have been studied and shown to be helpful. We also realize that there are many new products or therapies that have not been fully tested. The dozens of nonprescription "menopause formulas" found in health food stores or pharmacies attract millions of women seeking relief from "natural sources." The jury is out on many of these products. Although some women find relief with these products, some appear in studies to be ineffective; others can be dangerous if taken incorrectly or with other medications.

The challenge of any symptom relief plan is to improve your quality of life without increasing your risk for disease. If you consider medications, you need to carefully weigh the risks and benefits. Lifestyle approaches, on the other hand, can offer relief without risk and usually with substantial benefit. To help you in discussions with your clinician, we have gathered evidence on some of the latest treatments in both categories.

As you sift through this chapter, you'll see that we categorize by symptoms: hot flashes, PMS, mood changes, insomnia, and sexual and vaginal symptoms. Use this information as a guide. While these treatment options are not inclusive or intended to be recommendations, they do give you an idea of what women are trying, what's backed by scientific evidence and what is not. They should not re-place medical advice. Data change rapidly, so take the time to talk with your clinician about what's right for you—and keep asking.

Cooling Hot Flashes

Hot flashes are one of the toughest symptoms perimenopausal women cope with. While they are a real physical phenomenon, some-times external factors such as stress or caffeine can intensify them. So, we keep a woman's entire lifestyle in mind as we approach the man-agement of this symptom.

For Sonya, menopause was marked with night sweats. Like many women, this wasn't her only symptom, nor did it come at an easy time. For much of her adult life, she had enjoyed distance running, even running the length of the United States to promote well-being. But an old injury slowed her down and eventually put a stop to her running altogether. Sonya had considered running "a best friend," and the turn of events had left an emotional void. Night sweats and insomnia were now companions to her feelings of loss and sadness. "I think the menopause just heightened my inability to resolve this issue," she recalls. It was at this point that Sonya entered our pro-gram grieving the loss of running in her life and feeling powerless. The skills she learned helped her become more aware of her body and what she could do to control her symptoms.

One of the first things Sonya noticed about her night sweats was that alcohol was a trigger. She had never had this problem before, but she realized now that when she had alcohol, her body would react. In addition to limiting her triggers, she began to seek out new ap-proaches. In her words: "The first thing I did was acupuncture and that helped a lot. I started to incorporate soy into my diet. I was very strict with what I ate, which helped my sleep, helped the night sweats, and helped me emotionally." Sonya also maintained a modified exercise plan and began eliciting the relaxation response on a regular basis.

For Sonya it was about her entire way of life and knowing how to care for her body. She credits hot flash relief to her diet (including cutting back on alcohol) and, to some extent, to a renewed sense of empowerment that came from her proactive approach. "I think knowledge helped most—knowing that I could change, I could re-structure the way I thought about things. I felt empowered knowing that I could take control of my own health." How you manage hot flashes will depend on the degree to which they affect your life.

Mind/Body Approaches for Coping with Hot Flashes

Technique	Comment
Time	Symptoms will end naturally over time in most women, if you can wait them out.
Exercise	In one study, hot flashes were found to be half as common in physically active women compared to their sedentary counterparts. Although there is limited research on the exercise–hot flash link, the benefits of exercise on nearly every other body system should be reason enough to try it.
Avoid triggers	Pinpointing the things that trigger your hot flashes can be a giant step in reducing them. For many women, these include heat, hot drinks, spicy foods, alcohol, caffeine, and anger or stress. Reducing stress or avoiding other triggers during certain times of the day may help.

Keep cool
Dress in layers, so you can easily remove and replace clothes to adjust for hot flashes. With layers, you have more temperature control.

Understand your medications
Medications like tamoxifen (Nolvadex), used to treat breast cancer, and raloxifene (Evista), which is approved for prevention or treatment of osteoporosis, can cause hot flashes. Women taking these medications are not always aware of their side effects. Talk to your clinician about the medicines you take. Understanding how these medications affect hot flashes will help you know what to expect.

Relaxation techniques
Several studies show that relaxation techniques can provide significant relief. One of the pioneering researchers in this area, Robert Freedman, Ph.D., of Wayne State University in Detroit, found relaxation techniques involving deep-breathing exercises reduced self-reported hot flashes by about 50 percent. He teamed up with Suzanne Woodward, Ph.D., to test paced breathing exercises, muscle relaxation, and biofeedback. Objective skin temperature measurements helped conclude that the women who learned and practiced breathing techniques were able to reduce the number of hot flashes.

Creating a personal approach

What relieves hot flashes will vary from woman to woman. Some women, like Ann, will have a much tougher time. Ann was diagnosed

Mind/Body Approaches:
Paced Respiration (a.k.a. Minis)

Studies show that paced respiration practiced twice a day for fifteen minutes can help alleviate hot flashes. To try it, find a quiet area in which you can sit without too many distractions. Inhale slowly to the count of five and exhale slowly to the count of five, using diaphragmatic breathing. (See Chapter 3.) Once you master this technique, you can use it whenever you feel a hot flash coming on.

with invasive breast cancer, which has proved the battle of a lifetime. In addition to chemotherapy and the effects of induced menopause at age forty-two, she has also had to deal with the side effects of her medication—tamoxifen—which, while effective at treating breast cancer, often increases hot flashes.

Managing hot flashes has long been an issue for breast cancer patients. For this reason, the Mind/Body Medical Institute began a study to test an approach with no side effects or risks. In a randomized, controlled trial, women with tamoxifen-induced hot flashes were divided into two groups: the first received RR training and practiced daily for two months. The second, acting as a control group, did not receive any relaxation training. The RR group experienced significant reductions in the number of hot flashes. In this study, women who did not practice the RR demonstrated a significant increase in the intensity of their hot flashes.

Ann has found some relief through eliciting the relaxation response. Her hot flashes have become more tolerable because she has changed her approach in both mind and body. As a teacher, she used to dread hot flashes that would embarrass her in front of an entire classroom. Today, with a new perspective, she can find humor in it and has learned to dress in layers. "I've thrown away all my turtlenecks and have worked layering into my entire wardrobe. I've learned to peel like an onion. "

Considering Medication for Hot Flashes

If your hot flashes are causing insomnia and interfering with your life and you've tried lifestyle approaches without success, prescription drugs may be an attractive option. Ask yourself some questions as you consider this. What are the side effects? How would that drug interact with medications you already take? Talk with your clinician about the potential benefits and risks for you. The prescription medications listed are not intended to be recommendations or an inclusive listing. New medications continue to hit the market. And studies may change medical opinions. So, as in all cases, talk to your practitioner for detailed information.

Hormone therapy for hot flashes

The "level of evidence" (that is, the quality of the science that supports a treatment) for use of estrogen in reducing hot flashes is excellent. Many studies involving thousands of patients have consistently found that estrogen is very effective (80 to 90 percent reduction) for hot flash relief. With the exception of progestins (synthetic progesterone), nothing has proven as effective as estrogens. And while they are not recommended as long-term therapy to prevent disease, they are considered an appropriate short-term treatment for the alleviation of menopausal symptoms like hot flashes.

There are a variety of prescription products and doses to choose from. (See Chapter 7.) Many women and their clinicians prefer to start hormone therapy at the lowest possible dose, increasing only enough to ensure symptom relief. It's important to reexamine your estrogen use at regular intervals, taking into consideration your symptoms and new research findings. As mentioned, treatment of hot flashes for women with breast cancer can be particularly challenging. Estrogen, although the most effective way to control hot flashes, is considered potentially dangerous in this population, although no studies have been performed to establish this. Other gynecologic cancers (for example, of the uterus or ovaries) also raise concerns regarding the use of hormone therapy. In these cases, the appropriate treatment will depend on a variety of factors. Because risks and benefits are specific to the type of cancer, treatment is tailored for each patient.

Progestins: Progestins are hormones that act like natural progesterone in the body. A number of studies showed that progestins reduce hot flashes in a variety of patients. There are situations in which an estrogen may not be advised, for example, in a woman with a history of certain uterine cancers, but a progestin might be a desirable option. The long-term safety of progestin therapy has not been established.

Nonhormonal prescription medications to treat hot flashes

The weight of the evidence for the following prescription choices is not as strong as that for estrogen, although they are excellent alternatives for many women. When considering these options keep in mind that some of the studies were well done, but they have limitations. First, most of the trials included only a small number of participants so it is difficult to know if the same results would hold up in a larger sample. Second, many of the trials were of short duration and don't demonstrate whether a therapy would remain effective and safe over an extended period of time. Lastly, a number of the studies targeted specific populations of symptomatic postmenopausal women (such as breast cancer survivors) and these findings may not be true for all women.

Therapy	Comment
Antidepressants	If your doctor suggests an antidepressant medication for hot flashes, she is not implying that you are depressed. A number of antidepressants have preliminary data suggesting they work quite well for hot flashes.
	Effexor SR (venlafaxine): Initially developed as an antidepressant, it works both on serotonin and norepinephrine neurotransmitters. A study in breast cancer survivors showed a 45% decrease in hot flashes at a dose of 37.5 mg and a 60% decrease in hot flashes at a dose of 75 mg per day. The effects of venlafaxine occurred within a matter of days, compared with weeks for hormone therapy. At lower doses, side effects were minimal. At higher doses, some women may notice a dry mouth, decreased appetite, nausea, and constipation.
	Selective Serotonin Reuptake Inhibitors (SSRIs): This group of antidepressants including Prozac, Zoloft, and Paxil has shown some success in treating hot flashes. The long-term effects of these drugs are unknown. Pilot studies on several of the SSRI antidepressants demonstrated about a 40–50% reduction in hot flashes. They are more commonly used to treat PMS and depression. SSRIs can cause insomnia and adverse sexual side effects. As many as 30% or more of women report sexual side effects.
Neurontin (gabapentin)	An antiseizure medication initially developed for treatment of epilepsy shows great promise in re-

Therapy	Comment
	lieving hot flashes. A safe drug as prescription medications go, it has relatively few and mild side effects. A small study of breast cancer survivors showed a 66% reduction in hot flash frequency. A number of women in our program have also had success using this medication. In a study of fifty-nine women who experienced seven or more hot flashes per day, twelve weeks of gabapentin (900 mg per day) was associated with 45% fewer hot flashes. These women also reported a 54% reduction in hot flash composite score (an evaluation of hot flash frequency and severity combined into one measurement). Many women in our program report improved sleep with this medication.
Antihypertensives (blood pressure drugs)	Clinicians use Clonidine (Catapres) to treat high blood pressure (hypertension), and have prescribed it for hot flashes for some time. It is about 40–50% effective. While it may be useful for women with extreme hot flashes (such as the tamoxifen-induced hot flashes of breast cancer patients), its side effects may make it less than ideal for many women. These include headache, drowsiness, dry mouth, constipation, and insomnia.

Nonprescription therapies for hot flashes

There are many nonprescription products marketed as "natural" treatments" for menopause. If you choose an over-the-counter (nonprescription) dietary supplement, it's important to know that it is not FDA-regulated in terms of purity of content, dosage, or effectiveness. Many of these treatments have undergone only limited scientific studies involving small numbers and often in select patient populations. Thus, the science is inadequate to sufficiently assess their benefits or ultimate safety. Adding to the difficulty is the fact that placebo medications relieve hot flashes in 30 percent or more of women who take them. However, many clinicians as well as many menopause books strongly recommend various herbs and supplements. Some have had a long history of use in women. Often, patients are drawn to them because of this and because they seem natural and are more in line with their philosophies about health. The common questions are: "How do they work and are they effective?"

Ideally, there should be good scientific evidence for the supplements you use. Take caution when using any type of supplement. If you choose this route, it is often best to seek out the care of a practitioner with a special interest and training in complementary and alternative therapies. We will learn more as randomized clinical trials review these supplements. Until then, remember supplements carry untoward side effects, potential toxicity, and drug interactions just like prescription medications. Always talk to your practitioner about herbs and supplements you are taking. *And be sure to stop herbs and supplements two to three weeks before any surgeries or procedures.* The following show promise and are worthy of additional research:

Phytoestrogens: Phytoestrogens are plant estrogens found in soy, red clover (active ingredient called isoflavones), and flaxseed (called lignans.) A weak natural source of estrogen, soy has been touted as a woman's health cure-all. Some women swear by certain products, but the situation with soy has yet to be sorted out.

Because in countries like Japan, Korea, and China dietary consumption of soy is high, and the rate of menopausal symptoms low, researchers started to study this botanical for menopause-related symptoms. There is some evidence that eating soy foods such as tofu, in larger amounts, may help reduce hot flashes. A number of clinical trials have shown a 44–50 percent reduction, but other research has not been conclusive. In a review of eleven clinical trials that looked at soy or isoflavone supplements for hot flashes (products ranging from soy food to purified isoflavone preparations), only three of eight studies showed significant improvement in hot flashes at the end of the study. With regard to red clover isoflavones, studies have also been mixed with regard to effectiveness for menopausal hot flashes.

It is difficult to make accurate comparisons of soy research. The various studies have used different preparations (supplements or food), different doses and amounts of the active ingredients in soy, and were carried out for different lengths of time. What's more, menopausal symptoms often decreased in both treatment and placebo groups, so we really need better and longer studies to understand soy's true effects. There is also some uncertainty about soy's exact effect on breast tissue (see Chapter 6). Despite the lack of definitive data demonstrating hot flash benefits from soy, it is unlikely to be harmful to try including more whole soy foods into your diet. Many women report that soy helps them manage hot flashes. It has been a major part of many Asian diets and is presumed safe, though some women report upset stomachs. When considering soy, we suggest whole foods, and strongly recommend against pills or isolated extracts, which often contain high doses of isolated isoflavones. These have not been adequately studied, are not regulated or monitored for purity or safety, and there is no way to know for sure what you're getting. In addition, evidence shows many of the phytochemicals found in whole foods work in concert and when you extract the isoflavone from the protein there is little or no benefit. In the end, separating out one compound may leave you with a pill that has lost much of its potency and benefit.

Black cohosh: Black cohosh (*Cimicifuga racemosa*) has had a long history of use for menopausal symptoms. A century ago, women often turned to Lydia E. Pinkham's Vegetable Compound to ease "all those painful complaints so common to our best female population." Today, many of their great-granddaughters are using the compound's principle ingredient, black cohosh, for menopause relief.

It is one of the most common and most studied herbs found in over-the-counter menopause supplements. In Germany, where the German E Commission (similar to our FDA) regulates supplements, it is sold in a standardized form as Remifemin. Most of the studies have been done using this preparation. A recent review of randomized controlled trials of black cohosh reported a benefit for hot flashes in three out of four studies reviewed.

Side effects seem limited to mild gastric complaints, but high doses can produce headaches, vomiting, and dizziness. Anyone taking sedatives or tranquilizers should consult a physician before taking black cohosh. How black cohosh works is unknown. There is concern that it may pose a risk for women with breast cancer. So these women may be advised not to take black cohosh until more is known. Because no long-term safety studies exist, it is currently recommended that black cohosh not be taken for more than six months. If you're planning on taking black cohosh, we suggest using a product like Remifemin, which has a standardized dose.

Acupuncture

Steeped in thousands of years of Eastern tradition, and used for pain treatment, acupuncture has been gaining a following in Western medical circles for a variety of ailments. For the treatment of hot flashes, anecdotal evidence and a few pilot studies support the effectiveness of acupuncture in some women, although it is not completely risk free. If your state doesn't require a license to practice acupuncture, make sure that the practitioner you see is licensed in another state or certified by the National Certification Commission for Acupuncture and Oriental Medicine (www.nccaom.org). Many women find acupuncture relaxing and a perfect setting in which to elicit the relaxation response.

"Over-the-counter hormones": Over-the-counter "wild yam" creams are popular and promoted for menopausal symptoms. It is stated that the wild yam extract is either a precursor to producing hormones or aids the body in making hormones. Multiple health benefits are attributed, but there is no scientific data for these claims. The human body is not able to metabolize wild yam steroids. Furthermore, small placebo controlled, well designed studies showed no effect on menopausal symptoms.

Progesterone creams of various types are available over the counter but have not been well studied. One study suggests that the body doesn't absorb enough progesterone from the cream to have any effect on menopausal symptoms or provide other health benefits. Another study found that a progesterone cream was helpful in reduc-

The Herbal/Supplement Debate

Some herbs and supplements have claims that they can reduce hot flashes, but they don't always appear effective in studies. In well designed but small trials vitamin E, dong quai, ginseng, and evening primrose oil were found to be ineffective for hot flashes. However, a negative study is not necessarily the end of the story. There are several reasons for this: First, the correct "dose" is often unknown for a particular herb, and for some herbs there are multiple products of different potencies and origins. Second, many herbs, such as dong quai, would not necessarily be prescribed as a single agent by a practitioner of herbal therapy, and would more likely be incorporated into a mixture of herbs and other therapies. Clearly, significantly more research is needed on both the safety and effectiveness of herbal therapies for menopausal symptoms.

ing hot flashes. While more studies are warranted, remember that these products are not FDA regulated with regard to content, purity, or effectiveness.

Treating PMS and Mood Changes

Carrie's journey through perimenopause was plagued with insomnia; her mood was also affected. "I didn't know how to deal with menopause at all. I had a lot of emotional issues at the time. I feel like I wasn't myself. I was very stressed. I was anxious. My body didn't feel right. I was a mess. I didn't know what was happening to me."

PMS during perimenopause can be more severe and less predictable. PMS describes a constellation of symptoms that include depressed mood, anxiety, irritability, and mood swings as well as other physical symptoms. It occurs before the menstrual period, at which point symptoms typically go away for a period of time. The exact cause of PMS is unknown, but relates to the impact of rapidly changing ovarian hormone levels impacting brain neurotransmitters including, specifically, serotonin. "Perimenopausal PMS" has not been specifically studied, but is likely to respond to all of the therapies that work for regular PMS.

Lifestyle approaches

If you've ever used deep breathing to overcome anxiety or used a good workout to conquer anger, you may already know that the body has a chemical way of overcoming these powerful emotions. Both exercise and relaxation can help ease the emotional static of PMS. They are actually our top picks for getting out of a "blue mood."

Exercise, PMS, and mood: Virtually every study on exercise shows that it improves PMS. In addition, women with PMS who stop exercising tend to notice their PMS gets much worse. While the PMS and exercise studies are not randomized controlled trials, the overall health benefits of exercise combined with evidence for an improvement in PMS symptoms make it a first-line therapy for PMS.

A number of studies have shown that regular exercise can help lift depression. In fourteen controlled studies, aerobic exercise worked just as well as psychotherapy in treating mild to moderate depression. Besides relieving depression, exercise lessens anxiety and negative attitudes, and serves to boost self-esteem and life satisfaction.

The relaxation response: Stress has been correlated with increased severity of PMS symptoms. While at the Mind/Body Medical Institute, Harvard psychologist Alice Domar, Ph.D., attempted to test this hypothesis. Collaborating with her colleague Irene Goodale, Ph.D., she designed a study to determine whether utilizing the RR to decrease the body's response to stress would result in reduced severity of PMS. In her five-month study of 46 women with diagnosed severe PMS, the women were randomly assigned to three groups. In the first group, women charted their symptoms twice a day. In the second group, the women read leisure materials twice a day. Women in the third group listened to audiotapes to elicit the RR twice a day. At the end of five months, the women who practiced relaxation showed a 58 percent improvement in all PMS symptoms, compared to 27 percent improvement in the reading group and 17 percent improvement in the charting group.

Prescription therapies to address PMS and mood concerns

Selective serotonin reuptake inhibitors: SSRIs constitute the primary pharmacologic therapy for PMS. Two of these antidepressants (Sarafem and Zoloft) are currently approved for premenstrual dysphoric disorder (a severe form of PMS). Interestingly, these medications work very quickly (within a matter of days). Furthermore, women with PMS can take the medication only during the premenstrual time period and still get relief. (This is unlike the pattern seen in depressed patients who take these medications daily.) However, figuring out just when that premenstrual time period is can be difficult during perimenopause when cycles become irregular.

Estrogen: Can estrogen improve your mood? Some evidence suggests that estrogen has a positive effect on areas of the brain involved in the regulation of mood and behavior. And, in fact, estrogen has been shown to improve adverse mood symptoms, in particular, depressed mood in women during the perimenopause. This evidence is based on a few small studies.

GnRH agonists: These suppress hormone activity and induce a menopausal state. Because perimenopausal "PMS" improves after menstrual periods stop totally, a GnRH agonist, like Lupron, can be used to induce artificial menopause. This therapy is now used *less often* than SSRIs.

Nonprescription therapies

Over-the-counter remedies for PMS range from herbal remedies that can be dangerous to carbohydrate beverages. The good news is the options that are the safest appear effective.

Calcium carbonate: In a well-designed study 1,200 mg of calcium carbonate a day (example: Tums) was found to result in a 48 percent reduction of PMS symptoms (versus a 30 percent reduction in the placebo group). The symptoms the women were being scored on included negative mood, water retention, food cravings, and pain. The study found that all four symptom categories were significantly reduced three months after the women began taking the calcium. Because many American women have diets that are low in calcium, the use of calcium supplements actually can serve two purposes—potentially reducing symptoms and boosting calcium levels, which benefits the bones.

PMS Escape®: Certain carbohydrates may indirectly help the brain increase serotonin levels, which in turn would improve PMS. A controlled study found the carbohydrate-rich beverage PMS Escape to modestly improve symptoms, specifically depressed mood, anger, confusion, and carbohydrate cravings. It also appeared to improve memory word recognition.

Supplements/herbs: Many herbal "PMS formulas" have not been adequately studied. Various diets, vitamins, minerals, homeopathic remedies, and so on, are available, but most have no data from clinical trials to back up their claims or have studies with mixed results. The following supplements have not been studied specifically for perimenopausal symptoms or PMS, though they are widely marketed to menopausal women.

Headaches and Hormones

Hormonal changes have been linked with headaches. It's not uncommon to hear younger women complain of "menstrual migraines" around the time of their periods. The erratic hormonal fluctuations that precede menopause can make some perimenopausal women especially susceptible to migraines. Experts believe that changes in estrogen rather than a consistently low level may trigger migraines. For Becky, the splitting migraine headaches of perimenopause ended after menopause. Many women find their headaches get better or stop in the post-menopausal years.

Treatment depends on the cause and type of headache. Women say avoiding headache triggers, particularly when hormone levels are fluctuating, helps. Common headache triggers include alcohol, foods such as chocolate and aged cheeses, and stress. Talk with your clinician about medications that might help your type of headache. Some women find biofeedback or acupuncture to be helpful.

St. John's wort: Although St. John's wort has been used effectively to treat mild to moderate depression (not major depression), there have been no controlled studies supporting the use of St. John's wort specifically for perimenopausal symptoms.

Kava: There have been some claims that kava can help ease anxiety associated with perimenopause. *However,* kava has recently been linked to liver toxicity and liver failure. Because of this, Canada and countries in Europe have banned these supplements. The United States has issued warnings pending further studies regarding its safety.

Treating Insomnia

It has been well documented that we sleep less as we age. This is generally considered a normal part of the aging process. We also know that stress hormones, estrogen levels, the presence of hot flashes, and medical conditions that are more prevalent as we age all affect sleep patterns. The combination may explain why twice as many postmenopausal women as premenopausal women report sleep disturbances.

For Terry, as you may recall from Chapter 2, insomnia was about waking up early and not being able to fall back to sleep. This was followed by hours of racing thoughts and worry about not sleeping. Her solution involved improving her sleep hygiene (sleep habits) and a cognitive approach to restructure her thoughts about sleep. It also incorporated lifestyle adjustments and eliciting the relaxation response.

Sonya's case, waking up due to night sweats, is common among women at midlife. If you wake up at night in a drenching sweat, the effect on your sleep is obvious. Other hot flash–related temperature changes might not be so obvious. Although many women sleep through their hot flashes, at least one study showed that the most restorative form of sleep, known as REM, is still disrupted. Often

Lifestyle Approaches to Treating Insomnia

Approach	Comment
Break the cycle of insomnia	The following suggestions are taken from Dr. Gregg Jacobs's program:

Change habits: Cut out caffeine, alcohol, and nicotine, especially at night. Caffeine from a cup of coffee can take up to seven hours to clear your system. Alcohol can make you drowsy at first, but acts as a stimulant, often resulting in poor quality of sleep. Also, women metabolize alcohol more slowly as they age.

Restrict your sleep: A regular sleep schedule keeps the circadian sleep/wake cycle synchronized. Get up at about the same time every day, even after a late-night party or fitful sleep.

If you can't sleep, leave the bedroom: Go to bed only when you're sleepy. If you're unable to sleep, get up and move to another room. Stay up until you are sleepy, then return to bed. The idea is to train your body to associate your bed with sleep instead of sleeplessness and frustration.

Free yourself from worry: One idea Dr. Jacobs teaches is that nothing catastrophic happens if you don't sleep. This really helped Terry. She replaced her worry about not sleeping with thoughts of things that she could do at four o'clock in the morning. Terry's new attitude is "Why fight it? You can meditate; you can do a lot of other things. The biggest thing is not to make a big deal out of it." In particularly tough cases, medication may be suggested to break the insomnia cycle.

Elicit the relaxation response (RR)

The relaxation response itself can be used as an effective treatment for insomnia. Many women in our programs play their tapes, use guided imagery or a progressive muscle relaxation (see Chapter 3), and are amazed at how easily they drift off to sleep. Use a Walkman and reserve a specific tape or image to use only for sleep. The mind associates the voice or image with sleep and it will take less and less time to fall asleep as your body responds to the cue. (Remember that the physiologic benefits of RR are gained only after fifteen or twenty minutes have elapsed. So if you fall asleep before that, you will need to elicit the RR at an additional time during the day. Don't substitute a sleep-invoking RR "treatment" for a regular daily practice.)

Exercise

Physically active people sleep more soundly than their sedentary peers do. Aerobic exercise promotes restfulness by decreasing the time it takes to fall asleep, reducing the frequency of awakenings, and increasing deep sleep. Exercising five or six hours before bedtime encourages drowsiness when it's time to go to sleep, but be aware that exercising too close to bedtime can keep you awake.

when hot flashes are treated, sleep improves. Once Sonya controlled her night sweats, better sleep followed.

Because of its elusive and individual nature, the treatment of insomnia is beyond the scope of this book. But there are some basic approaches you might consider.

Lifestyle approaches to improve sleep

Barring underlying medical conditions, which should be discussed with your clinician, the treatment of choice for insomnia involves lifestyle changes. Many of our patients, including Terry, have found dramatic success following the Mind/Body Program for Insomnia, developed by Harvard psychologist and researcher Gregg Jacobs, Ph.D. The cognitive behavioral approaches he outlines in his book, *Say Goodnight to Insomnia,* involve changing beliefs about sleep, creating sleep "rituals," and incorporating cognitive and relaxation techniques. A careful evaluation can pave the way for better sleep by pinpointing habits that keep you up at night. From there, it's about changing the way you think.

Prescription treatments for insomnia

There are many prescription sleep aids hitting the market. Newer medications have fewer side effects. Still, this is an area that requires some consideration; you should consult with your clinician.

Women with severe hot flashes and night sweats naturally suffer from sleep disturbance and chronic sleep deprivation. In this situation, estrogen has been demonstrated to help with sleep. Natural progesterone also seems to help.

Nonprescription therapies to improve sleep

If you occasionally need help getting to sleep, you may be among the many who turn to over-the-counter (OTC) sleep medications. Unfortunately, those in search of sleep tend to overdo it, which may ulti-

Sweet Dreams at Midlife

With age come changes in sleep stages and reduced levels of chemicals such as melatonin and growth hormones that promote sleep. Maintaining healthy sleep habits can help. Here are some tips.

- Wake up and go to sleep at about the same time every day, even on weekends.
- Avoid caffeine or alcohol within three hours of bedtime.
- Exercise regularly; activity helps regulate the body's temperature systems. (Avoid exercise closer than three hours before bed. This can be a stimulant.)
- Stop smoking.
- Use the bed only for sleeping or sex.
- Relieve stress, depression, or anxiety with exercise or relaxation techniques. If sleep problems persist, psychotherapy or medication may help.
- Try to get as cool as possible before going to bed to help reduce night sweats.
- Seek treatment for conditions that compromise sleep (such as arthritis, congestive heart failure, sleep apnea, and hot flashes).

mately sabotage their efforts. One small survey of people age sixty and older found that more than a quarter had taken OTC sleeping aids in the preceding year—and one in twelve did so daily. Do these products work? Should you use them?

Be warned: Sleeping pills can promote sleep for a few nights but long-term use can actually worsen insomnia. Herbal supplements may be labeled "natural," but they contain biologically active substances that can have serious side effects. Unlike standard nonprescription sleeping pills, which contain a single antihistamine, many herbal products include a variety of active ingredients. Ask your clinician or pharmacist whether the ingredients might interact with other medications you may be taking.

Numerous herbs and supplements have been touted as being good for sleep, often without supporting evidence. Herbs such as

Insomnia and Medications

Not getting sleep? Are your medications the culprit? Sometimes medications can make you sleepy during the day, thus affecting nighttime sleep patterns. Others can make you jittery and unable to sleep. The laundry list of sleep-disrupting drugs is long and includes antidepressants such as Prozac (fluoxetine) and Zoloft (sertraline). Many patients taking fluoxetine require a second medication to help them sleep. Other sleep-disrupting medications include corticosteroids, thyroid hormones (if dose is too high), heart medications, clonidine, and a variety of others. Review your medications with your doctor to see if any of them could be interfering with your sleep.

chamomile and lavender have not been well studied, but women report that they're soothing. There are data that suggest valerian can help with insomnia. It may cause headaches, excitability, and heart irregularities. Melatonin is a popular sleep aid. Although it has been shown to be useful for easing jet lag, there are no good studies related to menopausal symptoms or age related insomnia. Potential side effects include morning-after headaches, increased risk of constricted blood vessels (women with heart problems should especially beware), and, in high doses, inhibited fertility. There is no data on long-term safety.

Treating Sexual and Vaginal Symptoms

The popularity of Viagra emphasizes the reality that sexuality remains very much a part of our lives as we age. The push for new products (ranging from lubricants to libido boosters) reminds us that there are many ways to deal with an age-old problem. But there is still that ancient, mystical, and largely unknown issue of desire.

As we focus on the mechanics of sex, we must remember that it is based on the deepest of emotions. (See Chapter 2.) Thus, we must pay attention to both the body and the mind when addressing issues of sexuality. How we feel about our partners, our lifelong attitudes about sexuality, our stress level, depression, and prescription medications all come into play. Furthermore, we don't fully understand what role menopause specifically plays in sexual desire.

The reality is, we have more questions than answers about sex hormones and their effects on sexuality. Some of the physical changes linked to these hormones are clear (see Chapter 2), but their impact on libido is not. Part of the complexity lies in the fact that some of the effects produced by hormones inside your body (biological effects) are not necessarily the same as those produced from a pill form (pharmacological effects). Research on effective treatments is ongoing. While there are a variety of treatments available to address the physical aspects of sexuality, a mind/body approach also relies on nurturing the emotional aspects of intimacy.

If you are having difficulties, one of the first steps is to have an open discussion with your clinician. Naturally, this isn't always easy. Many clinicians do not ask about sexual issues. So you may have to initiate the conversation. Here are some issues you might expect him or her to discuss with you in a sensitive, confidential, and nonjudgmental manner:

- Your medical history
- Any existing depression or anxiety
- Sexual function (of you and your partner) and relationship issues
- Risks and benefits of potential medications, including hormones
- A referral to a specialist, if needed

A physical exam, including a pelvic exam, can evaluate vaginal health and will pinpoint any physical problems. Your provider may include lab tests such as an FSH level; thyroid tests; and possibly free testosterone (most testosterone in the blood is bound to a protein and therefore is biologically inactive; a "free" testosterone test measures the amount of unbound, and therefore active, testosterone in the bloodstream), although this is controversial.

Vaginal dryness

Vaginal pain is a common complaint in postmenopausal women. Estrogen is directly linked to protecting vaginal tissue. Decreased lubrication is related to declining estrogen levels and can lead to vaginal dryness. These and other physical changes related to menopause (see Chapter 2) can result in irritation and pain. This, in turn, can have a dampening effect on libido. The good news is that there are a variety of effective treatments available. These include lubricants, vaginal moisturizers, and vaginal estrogens.

Lubricants: Lubricants are slippery substances that can be used at the time of intercourse. Most vaginal lubricants are available without a prescription. Popular water-based lubricants include such products as Lubrin and KY Personal Lubricant.

Vaginal moisturizers: Vaginal moisturizers contain a compound that adheres to the vaginal wall and draws in the body's moisture. They can be used twice weekly on a regular basis (unlike lubricants, which are applied at the time of intercourse). Examples of vaginal moisturizers include Replens and KY Long Lasting Vaginal Moisturizer.

Estrogen creams: Vaginal estrogen creams are highly effective in relieving vaginal dryness and painful intercourse. However, the estrogen in these creams is easily absorbed into the circulation. So unless a woman has had a hysterectomy (removal of the uterus), she may also need some form of progesterone to avoid precancerous changes in the uterus. Even though vaginal estrogen creams are absorbed, the doses are generally low. Thus, women can gain relief without some of the risks associated with systemic hormone therapy.

Estrogen rings: Another locally applied product is a ring containing estradiol (Estring) that is inserted into the vagina much like a diaphragm. The ring releases a low dose of estrogen that has very little systemic absorption. The ring is replaced every three months. Some oncologists have allowed breast cancer survivors to use the Estring ring because very little of the estrogen reaches the bloodstream. Over short periods of time, the ring seems to be safe without progesterone, but long-term studies are lacking. Some clinicians recommend that all women with a uterus who use estrogen in any form take progesterone as well.

Estrogen tablets: Estrogen tablets (Vagifem) can be inserted into the vagina with an applicator to relieve vaginal symptoms. Similar to the above methods, they won't help systemic symptoms such as hot flashes, and if a woman has a uterus, progesterone may be recommended.

Once vaginal dryness is successfully treated, it can pave the way for more comfortable and enjoyable sex. And the irony is . . . regular sexual stimulation can help maintain vaginal elasticity. In fact, it is recommended as a treatment. During intercourse, masturbation, and foreplay, blood flow to the vaginal area increases. This improves lubrication and supports the health of the vagina.

Desire, arousal, and orgasm

There are many factors that determine our sexuality. While estrogen is a major hormonal player, androgens (including testosterone and other hormones called DHEAs) likely play a role in female sexuality. For women, it is important to remember that sexual interest is often triggered by a desire for intimacy more than the satisfaction of sexual urges. A broader mind/body approach to this uncharted and often confusing territory would embrace all of these biologic, psychological, cultural, interpersonal, and individual factors.

Combating Urinary Incontinence

Over the years, pelvic floor muscles weaken. For some women, this can lead to urinary incontinence. Up to 30 percent of American women aged fifty to sixty-four have problems with this. Fear of embarrassment can prompt women to avoid sex altogether. If you're having a problem with incontinence, talk with your clinician. Although sometimes a difficult issue to bring up, it should be discussed, because it is treatable. There are a variety of medications, procedures, and devices that can help. There are also ways to exercise your pelvic floor muscles to help prevent it. Strengthening these muscles can actually improve conditions like urinary incontinence, while enhancing sexual pleasure.

You can strengthen pelvic floor muscles with an exercise invented in the 1950s by Dr. Arnold Kegel. Known as "Kegels," the exercise is simple and can be done anywhere:

1. Locate your pelvic floor muscles by pretending to stop the flow of urine while urinating. Alternatively, you can contract the anal sphincter as you would to prevent bowel movement. You will feel a distinct tightening of your muscles.
2. Tighten these muscles again, hold for ten seconds, and then release. Repeat this ten times.
3. Repeat five to ten times each day.

Estrogen: Declining estrogen may affect sexual desire and arousal because this hormone influences blood flow and the nervous system. Data from the Melbourne Women's Midlife Health Study support this idea. It found that lower blood estrogen levels were linked with lowered sexual arousal and libido. In postmenopausal women, studies show that estrogen therapy restores genital sensation close to the levels in premenopausal women, and that it can also improve blood flow to the vaginal area.

Androgens: Although often thought of as "male hormones," androgens (including testosterone) are important for women as well. They likely play a role in maintaining sexual desire, muscle mass, bone density, fat distribution, mood, energy, and feelings of well-being. Unlike estrogen, they do not dramatically decline with natural menopause, but do decline with induced or surgical menopause.

Some experts have described an "androgen insufficiency syndrome," which is marked by low androgen levels, a persistent sense of fatigue and low energy, changes in sexual interest and function, and an overall diminished sense of well-being. Diagnosing such a deficiency requires an evaluation by your gynecologist.

Treatments for female sexual dysfunction

Most women note some changes in sexuality as they pass through menopause. If significant changes in your "sexual self" upset you, talk with your clinician. Sexual dysfunction is a catchall phrase for a variety of highly complex issues such as less desire for sex, difficulty becoming sexually "aroused," or changes in your ability to have an orgasm. If these problems are subtle or they don't bother you, then it's not a case of sexual dysfunction.

Female sexual dysfunction is an area of intense research and debate. Few treatments are FDA approved for female sexual dysfunction, but products are being prescribed. Again, your best bet is to get as much information as possible and review risks and benefits with your clinician.

EROS device: The EROS device is a hand-held, battery-operated clitoral suction device. The vacuum stimulates the clitoral area and increases blood flow and engorgement. This is FDA approved for female sexual dysfunction, specifically for problems with arousal.

Testosterone: Some women with low sexual desire may benefit from testosterone replacement. There is no FDA-approved testosterone product; however, there is an estrogen plus synthetic testosterone product called Estratest. This combination therapy has been found to improve a number of quality of life symptoms, including sexual dysfunction, in surgically menopausal women. It is intended for use in women whose hot flashes are not responding to estrogen, but clinicians also prescribe it for women with low testosterone levels following removal of their ovaries.

In 2000, researchers from nine medical centers across the country tested an experimental testosterone skin patch. They reported that a lower testosterone dose—one designed to bring women's testosterone levels more in line with the premenopausal norm—improved sexual response without adverse effects. They studied seventy-five healthy women who said that their sexual pleasure had declined after their ovaries were removed. All were taking estrogen and all were in stable, long-term heterosexual relationships.

The women wore three different skin patches—one with an inactive substance (placebo), one with 150 mcg of testosterone, and one with 300 mcg of testosterone—for twelve weeks each. At the end of the study, the researchers found that when the women were on the higher testosterone dose, they had sex more often and enjoyed it more. The lower dose also helped, but to a lesser degree, as did the inactive patch. The researchers suggest that the women's desire to improve their sex lives may have powered this placebo effect. It's also possible that in women who took testosterone first, their patterns of sexual activity while taking testosterone carried over into the placebo phase of the study. Research is now under way on "naturally" menopausal women with low sexual desire.

Some clinicians prescribe custom "compounded" testosterone preparations. (See Chapter 7.) These are not FDA approved or regulated. These products, including topical 2 percent testosterone cream or ointment, may be applied directly to the vagina and clitoral area (or any skin surface). Many women report improved libido; however, no controlled studies have confirmed this. Absorption is highly variable and safety has not been established.

Viagra: As of this wriing, Viagra (sildenafil) is not FDA approved for use in women and studies on its use in women have been mixed. It is likely that there are specific women that may benefit from Viagra. For example, a preliminary study showed Viagra to be helpful for women with SSRI-related sexual dysfunction. Further studies of Viagra for women are in progress.

Wellbutrin: Wellbutrin was initially designed as an antidepressant, and then later became well known as Zyban, the smoking cessation aid. A libido-enhancing effect of Wellbutrin has been suspected with limited data suggesting efficacy. In addition, Wellbutrin has also been effective for some women in countering SSRI-induced sexual dysfunction.

An assortment of new therapies: Over the next few years there will be an explosion of data and products for sexual dysfunction. Many of these will be initially tested in men with erectile dysfunction. However, a number will be evaluated for sexual dysfunction in women also. The products range from herbal therapies (like ArginMax for women), to amino acid/herb combinations (L-arginine and yohimbine). New Viagra-like drugs and other medications are in clinical trials. Again, talk with your clinician about the latest treatments and their side effects.

Communication and sexuality

Communication, understanding, and intimacy—all enhance and alter the sexual setting. If you are happy with your sex life or intimate bond, chances are you don't need advice. If you are interested in improving your sex life, talk with your partner about your mutual needs and expectations. Explore your own emotional inhibitions. Are there cultural messages or stereotypes that you can shed? Body image, self-esteem,

Strategies for Improving Libido

- Allow more time for manual or oral stimulation.
- Experiment with erotic materials, sexual fantasies, vibrators, dildos.
- Try a mindful/sensual massage or a warm bath.
- Change the sexual routine: location, time of day.
- Use vaginal lubricants (water-based).
- Explore noncoital sexual activity, such as oral sex or mutual masturbation.
- Communicate with your partner about sexual or other concerns.
- Check your medicine cabinet. (More than two hundred medications have sexual dysfunction as a side effect. Check with your doctor about switching to another drug that does not have sex-related side effects: there often are such options for you.)

Adapted from *Treatment Strategies for Improving Libido,* North American Menopause Society, Core Curriculum Guide.

and trust in a partner all might be addressed. If talking is too difficult, counseling with a trained sex therapist can help pave the way.

For many women, opening up and talking about sex is the first step in a rewarding journey. Many popular books on midlife explore the concept of "a wild woman" within. This concept (and mind-set) encourages women to be creative and to let their true selves come forth. We encourage this mind-set in regard to your sexuality. Try experimenting and explore new ways to honor your sexuality and needs for intimacy. (See Chapter 4.) Be creative, practice mindfulness, and cultivate joy in the process.

Often increasing the bonds between partners will help shift the focus from any physical limitations. In the end, intimacy and a good relationship with your partner may be the best therapy. "What's love got to do with it?" Apparently, quite a bit.

Protecting Your Health: Heart Disease, Osteoporosis, Breast Cancer, and Alzheimer's Disease

A s we age, we grow wiser. We have journeyed many miles and laughed many times through our first four or five decades. And the second half of life can prove just as rewarding, if not more so. The key to embracing midlife and beyond involves staying healthy and that means taking a proactive approach to protecting your health.

Many women are concerned that they may be at high risk for disease once they reach menopause. This is a confusing realm. On one hand, some diseases like osteoporosis and heart disease have been linked to menopause. On the other hand, they are also linked to aging. There is a general belief that the natural estrogen a woman produces through her childbearing years protects certain systems like the heart and the bones. However, the exact role of estrogen remains a mystery. We know that estrogen helps protect bone. Circulating naturally in a woman's body, it has been thought to have a protective effect on the heart. It's believed to relax artery walls and alter the production of proteins in the liver that influence cholesterol levels in the blood (tending to lower LDL and increase HDL). Because there are estrogen receptors throughout a woman's body, it is possible that estrogen naturally circulating also benefits other parts of the body like the brain. However, supplementing hormones after menopause, as we have learned, is not a simple switch.

As you think about reducing your risk for disease remember that estrogen is just one piece of a very complex puzzle. Your overall health and risk for disease are determined by many factors. In this chapter, we take a mind/body approach to help you reduce your risk for those diseases that become more common in the years after menopause. Our message: you can control how you age.

Protecting Your Heart

Heart disease is the most common disease and the number one cause of death in women. Surveys show that women are most fearful of dying of breast cancer, yet they're ten times more likely to develop heart disease and six times more likely to die from it. The traditional male hallmark symptom, severe chest pain, can be missing in a woman. She might instead complain of overwhelming fatigue; shortness of breath; nausea; indigestion; dizziness; back discomfort; or a pain or tingling in the arm, neck, or jaw.

Heart disease is uncommon in premenopausal women. However, after menopause, when estrogen levels drop, the risk for heart disease increases, particularly after the age of sixty-five. Despite this fact, the relationship between heart disease, menopause, and estrogen is unclear and the subject of intense debate and research. Many changes take place as we age, not all of them related to estrogen. The following are heart disease risk factors:

- Smoking
- Lack of physical activity
- Obesity
- High blood pressure
- Abnormal cholesterol levels
- Diabetes mellitus
- Elevated blood levels of a natural substance called C-reactive protein (or CRP)
- Elevated blood levels of another natural substance called homocysteine
- Family member with heart attack or stroke. For women, risk is increased if they have a mother or sister who developed coronary artery disease before sixty-five years old, or if their father or brother developed coronary artery disease before fifty-five years old.
- Race: black
- Advancing age
- Postmenopausal status (early menopause can increase risk)

Some of us are genetically at higher risk for heart disease. Fortunately, even if—for example—we have a family member with heart disease, we can take steps to prevent it in ourselves. The truth is, there is a great deal you can do to reduce your risk. Remember this:

- More heart disease can be prevented by lifestyle modification than by any medicine that a doctor can prescribe. By increasing your exercise, achieving a healthy weight, and stopping smoking you can do more to protect yourself against heart disease than any pill available.

- Your doctor can help, particularly if you have a condition like high blood pressure or high cholesterol that can be treated with medicines. But you can do more for yourself, with lifestyle changes, than any clinician can do for you.
- The converse is also true. No matter how hard your clinician works to protect you against heart disease, if you do not adopt a healthy lifestyle your doctor's help may not be enough.

Preventing heart disease

There are a growing number of ways to predict heart disease. There are also important screenings and treatments that can prevent problems before they occur.

New cholesterol targets: Monitoring your cholesterol levels is a proven way to predict your risk. In 2002, the National Institutes of Health issued new guidelines for cholesterol testing and management. It recommended a more comprehensive fasting lipid profile, which measures not only total cholesterol, but LDL cholesterol, HDL cholesterol, and triglycerides. Each of these has been found to be an independent risk factor for heart disease. And clinicians now interpret these results in the context of your overall heart disease risk. (See Chapter 6 for newer cholesterol guidelines.)

Cholesterol-lowering drugs: There are many cholesterol-lowering drugs that may be prescribed alone or in combination. Statins (reductase inhibitors) are the newest, most widely used class of cholesterol-lowering drugs. They work by changing the way the liver processes fats in the blood (lipids). In effect, they restrict the amount of cholesterol that can be deposited into the bloodstream and increase the amount of LDL (bad cholesterol) that can be carried out of the bloodstream. Large, randomized clinical trials have shown that people who use statins have a 20–30 percent reduction in death from heart disease and in the incidence of major cardiovascular events, such as heart attacks, strokes, and angina (chest pain due to insufficient blood flow to the heart muscle). Statins have few known side effects, but in rare cases they have caused damage to the liver and muscles. Your clinician may monitor you with blood tests early in treatment, and should make you aware of the symptoms that suggest these problems. Whether or not you should take a statin depends on your lipid profile, other risk factors, medications, and general health.

Selective estrogen receptor modulators (SERMs): There has been an increased focus on the role of SERMs (selective estrogen receptor modulators) for heart health as well as bone health. Raloxifene (Evista) has been shown to decrease levels of both LDL and fibrinogen (part of the blood-clotting process), which can lower cardiovascular risk. Unlike estrogen, raloxifene doesn't elevate levels of triglycerides or C-reactive protein, both risk factors for heart disease in women. An analysis of raloxifene use in osteoporotic women showed a reduction in cardiovascular events in women assessed to be at high risk for heart disease. Additional data are expected to shed more light on the potential role of SERMs in managing heart disease.

The pros and cons of aspirin: Randomized trials have provided clear evidence of aspirin's value in both preventing and treating cardiovascular diseases. Overall, dozens of studies involving tens of thousands of people have shown that low-dose aspirin reduces the risk for heart disease and stroke by about 25 percent. Based on these and other findings, investigators speculate that giving aspirin to a patient within hours of a heart attack might also be beneficial. Despite aspirin's benefits, it also has some drawbacks. It can increase the risk for brain hemorrhage and gastrointestinal bleeding. So, should you be taking aspirin? How do you weigh the benefits and the risks? In 2002, the U.S. Preventive Services Task Force addressed these questions. After reviewing five large, ongoing studies of heart disease prevention, the task force concluded that aspirin would likely benefit people who didn't have heart disease but were at high risk for coronary artery disease or heart attack. However, it recommended that people at low risk for heart disease not take aspirin because of possible side effects, such as gastrointestinal bleeding.

Heal the heart from within

The heart is considered the center of the soul as well as the organ that keeps blood flowing throughout the body. Could it be that our minds and emotions influence the heart, beyond the Valentine's Day metaphors? Medical science is proving that psychological influences are literally heartfelt, and can contribute to cardiac risk. Psychological stress, anger, social isolation, and depression appear to raise the risk for coronary artery disease and the risk of dying after a heart attack. Stress may also affect triglyceride levels. If hostility and anger are issues for you, seek counseling and learn new ways of releasing tension. Many of the RR skills in this and our cardiac book *Mind Your Heart* are designed to address these very issues.

Adopting a heart-smart lifestyle

Many of the techniques that can make your experience of menopause as positive as possible will also improve your health in many ways. But it is hard to incorporate changes into a busy life! Talk of exercising, losing weight, and kicking bad habits like smoking are sometimes lost to fatigue after a long day. But, keep in mind that a few changes can rival the best medications.

If you have heart disease, are at high risk for it, or simply want to know more about managing it, we suggest you read *Mind Your Heart*. It's based on the teachings of our Mind/Body Cardiac Wellness Program. We have been fortunate at the Mind/Body Medical Institute to watch patients in our Cardiac Wellness Program turn their lives and their risk factors around. After improving lifestyle behaviors and learning methods to cope better with stress, patients have lowered cholesterol and blood pressure levels, reduced medical symptoms, and increased their capacity for exercise.

Protecting Your Bones

It is true that bone loss accelerates after menopause. But it is also a fact that not all women will have problems. How do you avoid those problems? There are some bone-building facts that can help.

Many people assume bones are solid masses, concrete in nature. After all, they do have the strength to carry us through life. But bone is actually living tissue that is constantly being broken down ("resorbed") and rebuilt. This process of resorption and formation is called "remodeling" and involves a balance between "builders" (osteoblasts) and "destroyers" (osteoclasts). One of the essential building blocks of this process is calcium. Calcium is also crucial for the proper function of other parts of the body including the heart, brain, and nervous systems. When we don't get enough calcium in our diets, the bones sacrifice their calcium to support other parts of the body. As we age, we have a tougher time absorbing calcium from our diets. This combination contributes to the loss of bone health, but it is not the only factor. As we get older, the dismantling of bone outpaces the building of bone. Declining estrogen levels have an immediate impact on bone health because estrogen plays a critical role in slowing bone loss. The dramatic decline in estrogen associated with menopause triggers an imbalance (rate of loss greater than formation) that speeds bone loss in the years following menopause.

Osteoporosis and risk for fracture

Osteoporosis is characterized by low bone mass and reduced bone quality, resulting in increased fracture risk. Fractures are the biggest

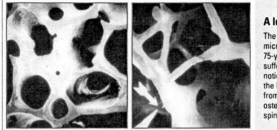

A look at osteoporotic bone
The photograph at left shows a microscopic view of bone from a 75-year-old woman who does not suffer from osteoporosis. You'll notice that her bone is denser than the bone shown at right, which is from a 47-year-old woman with osteoporosis who has had several spinal fractures.

problem associated with osteoporosis. Often osteoporosis is a "silent disease" until that first fracture. Fractures pose a serious health threat and can lead to loss of independence for both men and women. An estimated 10 million Americans have bones porous enough to warrant the diagnosis, and some experts consider bone loss and hip fracture to be at epidemic proportions in people over sixty-five.

When fractures do occur, they can be devastating, particularly hip fractures in an older person. As many as 24 percent of hip fracture patients over age fifty die within a year. An additional 25 percent will require long-term care, and 50 percent will have some long-term loss of mobility. At six months after a hip fracture, only 15 percent of hip fracture patients can walk across a room unaided. This can literally mean moving from independence to long-term care in a nursing home with one fall! The resulting lack of mobility also puts patients at great risk for a second fracture. Balance, strength, bone density, lifestyle choices, even the placement of furniture, all affect a woman's fracture risk.

Risk factors for osteoporosis

Osteoporosis is of particular concern for all women as they get older. First, compared with men, women have less bone tissue. The drop in estrogen following menopause causes us to lose the bone mass we do have faster. Second, for both women and men, aging causes bones to become weaker. The older you are, the greater your risk. Certain circumstances can further increase the chances that you will develop osteoporosis. The National Osteoporosis Foundation points to the following as risk factors:

- Breaking a bone after age fifty
- Current low bone mass
- History of fracture in a first-degree relative (mother or sister, for example)
- Being thin and/or having a small frame
- A family history of osteoporosis
- Low estrogen levels due to menopause—especially if you experienced menopause early or had your ovaries removed
- Abnormal absence of menstrual periods
- Anorexia
- Low lifetime calcium intake
- Certain medications, such as prednisone and anticonvulsants
- An inactive lifestyle
- Current cigarette smoking
- Excessive use of alcohol
- Race—Caucasian and Asian women are at increased risk, although African Americans and Hispanic Americans are at significant risk as well

There is a clear link between low estrogen, osteoporosis, and fracture risk. Yet, like heart disease, there are many things you can do to maintain bone strength, balance, and health.

We achieve peak bone mass in our twenties and thirties and then begin to gradually lose it. Our peak bone mass is genetically determined. How much bone we ultimately build, however, depends on lifestyle. Diet is critical, which is why it's so important for teens to pay attention to calcium intake. Reaching peak bone mass when you're young means you have more of a buffer later in life when bone loss is a concern. Bone building is a continual process; it's never too

Stress and Your Bones

While stress is not typically considered a risk factor for osteoporosis, there is evidence it may impact your bones. Cortisol, one of the key "stress" hormones, has been found to suppress bone formation and decrease calcium absorption. In her book, *Strong Women, Strong Bones,* Miriam Nelson describes a 1996 study published in the *New England Journal of Medicine* that explored a possible link between depression and bone health. This study looked at twenty-four pairs of women aged thirty to forty. The women matched each other in weight and nutritional status. However, one member of each pair had a history of depression, while the other did not. Those who were depressed had less bone density. There is a chance that depressed women exercise less. So, while the study does not prove a link, it is definitely food for thought.

late to start. In addition to diet (Chapter 6), weight bearing exercises like walking and strength training (Chapter 5) all put pressure on bones, which helps make them stronger.

Measuring bone density

The best approach to osteoporosis is to prevent it. If you already have it, the goal of management is to prevent a fracture. Both involve monitoring your bone health. Bone mineral density (BMD) testing is the most effective method for determining a fracture risk. This screening measures your bone's mineral content. In general, the lower your bone density, the higher your risk for fractures.

There are several tests that assess bone mass. The gold standard of BMD testing is the dual-energy X-ray absorptiometry (DXA). This technique can measure BMD at any spot in the body. It is most often used to measure bone density at the hip and spine. The process is quick, taking only ten minutes. And it's simple. A patient lies on a table while the imager passes over the body. It uses only one-tenth of the radiation exposure of a standard chest X ray. The downside to this DXA is that it requires sophisticated machinery, usually found in a hospital radiology department. Not every community will have DXA testing readily available.

The push is on to prevent osteoporosis, which means screening more women who may be at risk. While it is most commonly diagnosed in slender, postmenopausal white women, other populations would benefit from screening. Osteoporosis in Hispanic women appears to be higher than once believed. And while African American women are considered at a lower risk, there still may be 300,000 African American women who are at risk. Today, there is a push to expand screening to serve larger patient populations. All women over age sixty-five and younger postmenopausal women with risk factors can benefit from bone density screening.

Ultrasound, which uses sound waves to measure bone at the heel, is increasingly available in places where DXA isn't practical or available. Ultrasound does not give measurements like those provided by DXA, but it seems to predict fracture risk. Quick, compact, lightweight, and easy to use, the sonometer is already in use at many medical facilities, and may soon turn up in physicians' offices and even pharmacies.

BMD scoring: To decide what levels place people at risk, statisticians looked at the bone densities of thousands of women and noted who had osteoporotic fractures and who didn't. Since women who are in their thirties (when bone mass is at its peak) have the lowest fracture risk, their average bone mass was used as the reference point. Osteoporosis is defined in terms of standard deviations from the average peak bone mass, also called a T-score. Standard deviation is a statistical term used to express the amount of variation away from the mean or average.

A finding of low bone mass (osteopenia) is not reason for alarm. It does *not* mean you will have osteoporosis or that you are at great

Understanding Bone Mineral Density Results

If your T-score is:	
Greater than −1	Your bone density is considered normal.
−1 to −2.5	You do not have osteoporosis but do have osteopenia (low bone mass), which is not a disease.
−2.5 or less	You have osteoporosis, even if you haven't broken a bone.

risk for fractures. Women with a diagnosis of osteopenia should talk with their clinicians. The best approach is an individualized one that takes into account a woman's particular risk factors and the potential benefits of any proposed treatment plan.

Reducing fracture risk

For older people, fractures can have devastating consequences, including significant disability and even death. Most osteoporosis-related fractures occur in one of three sites: the hips, the vertebrae, or the wrists. Regardless of your bone density, the biggest risk factor for a fracture is a prior fracture. So, preventing that first fracture is critical. That's why so much emphasis is placed on predicting fracture risk. While bone mineral density tests can help gauge your risk, they aren't the only predictors. Some women can have low bone density but not have fractures. Other factors that can increase your chance of falling and breaking a bone include:

- Low levels of physical activity
- Low muscle mass or impaired strength
- Balance problems
- Poor eyesight

- Medications, such as sedatives and blood pressure drugs, that can cause dizziness, lightheadedness, or impaired balance
- A history of falls
- Environmental hazards, such as electrical cords or throw rugs in walking paths
- Advanced age

Preventing and treating bone loss

The foundation for prevention and treatment is simple. Get enough calcium and vitamin D, engage in weight-bearing exercise regularly, and take appropriate medications when necessary. Your diagnosis and treatment will involve evaluating your risk factors and current health status. If you determine you are at risk, there are a number of medications your clinician will discuss with you.

Bisphosphonates: Many women take bisphosphonates to preserve bone density. Two commonly prescribed bisphosphonates are alendronate (Fosamax) and risedronate (Actonel). They both are available in a once-a-week dose. Unlike hormone therapy, they do not have any beneficial (or negative) estrogenic effects. Both have excellent studies demonstrating prevention of vertebral and hip fractures in women with osteoporosis. New bisphosphonates, including a once-a-year version, are in development. Bisphosphonates are generally tolerated well by most people who take them. To avoid problems like irritation of the esophagus and stomach (digestive tract) it is recommended they be taken with a full glass (6–8 ounces) of plain water on an empty stomach first thing in the morning while remaining upright.

Calcitonin (Miacalcin): Unlike the other bisphosphonate medications mentioned, calcitonin is approved only for the *treatment,* not the prevention, of osteoporosis. Generally, calcitonin is regarded as a less effective treatment because it doesn't build bone as robustly as other medications, and it is unclear whether it helps prevent hip or wrist fractures. Although it is a relatively weak bone-builder, calcitonin may offer a unique benefit: some people have reported that it relieved their bone pain. So it is sometimes prescribed for people who have significant pain following vertebral fractures. Side effects of calcitonin (taken in the form of a nasal spray) are minimal.

Hormone therapy: Hormone therapy remains an excellent bone drug. Because of its risks, if osteoporosis is your primary concern, you will be advised to find an alternative. However, if you're taking HT for quality of life reasons, it will also benefit your bones.

Estrogen is most effective in retarding bone loss when therapy begins shortly after the onset of menopause. While it may be able to stave off some bone loss early on with short-term use, once it is discontinued, its bone benefits are lost over time.

Selective estrogen receptor modulators and bones: SERMs, or "designer" estrogens, as they are often called, have generated a great deal of interest because they are designed to exert beneficial estrogenic effects in some areas of the body, like the bones, and yet have anti-estrogenic activity in other parts of the body, such as the uterus or breast. Raloxifene (Evista) is one of the selective estrogen receptor modulators. Like estrogen, raloxifene slows bone loss, but it does not increase the risk for uterine cancer, and it seems to protect against breast cancer as well.

In a major clinical trial designed to evaluate raloxifene's effects on osteoporotic fractures (the Multiple Outcomes of Raloxifene Evaluation, or MORE), more than 7,000 women with osteoporosis took either raloxifene or placebo and were followed for three years. The reduction in vertebral fractures among those taking raloxifene was similar to that observed with alendronate (Fosamax). In contrast to bisphosphonates, raloxifene does not have data demonstrating reduction in hip fractures.

There are other possible health benefits of raloxifene, specifically breast cancer prevention and lower rates of heart disease, that are under investigation. During the MORE trial, raloxifene reduced the risk for breast cancer by 76 percent and also reduced the risk of heart disease in high-risk women. Side effects included hot flashes and deep vein thrombosis, a condition causing blood clots in deep veins, most commonly in the legs. There are currently a number of additional SERMs in development.

Parathyroid hormone (PTH): In the body, the parathyroid glands produce this hormone, which ensures the proper balance of calcium. Recombinant human parathyroid hormone (an artificial form of PTH) stimulates bone formation and builds bone. It is a very effective treatment for osteoporosis and causes significant increases in bone density. For postmenopausal women who have suffered vertebral fractures, PTH lowers the risk of future fractures by 50–70 percent. PTH is taken by daily injection. In 2003, the FDA approved a form of PTH called teriparatide (Forteo) specifically for the treatment of osteoporosis.

Breast Cancer

Breast cancer is most common in women over age fifty and it has been linked to the long-term use of hormone therapy. For these and many other reasons, it is a major concern for menopausal women.

Risk factors for breast cancer

To be at risk for breast cancer means having a greater likelihood of developing the disease. Unfortunately, the elusive nature of cancer makes understanding risk factors a bit tough. Having one or more risk factors does not mean you will get the disease. At the same time, having no risk factors does not protect you from it.

In addition to being female, the following are some of the known risk factors:

- Personal history of breast, ovarian, endometrial, or colon cancer
- Mother or sister with breast cancer
- Getting your first period before age twelve; late menopause
- Never having had a baby; first baby after age thirty
- Lifestyle: lack of exercise; alcohol; diet low in fruits and vegetables
- Radiation exposure: women who have had chest area radiation treatment earlier have a greatly increased risk of breast cancer (example: Hodgkin's disease)
- Long-term use of hormone therapy

Gender: Both women and men develop breast cancer, but it is more common in women, largely because their breasts undergo a complex hormonal evolution as they mature during their teens and early twenties and are exposed to cycling hormones during their menstrual years.

Age: The chance of getting this disease rises sharply as a woman gets older. Breast cancer chiefly occurs in women who are over fifty and it's uncommon in women under thirty-five.

Family medical history: Vulnerability to breast cancer is heightened for any woman who has a close blood relative diagnosed with the disease. Having one first-degree relative (mother, sister) with breast cancer approximately doubles a woman's risk. Having two first-degree relatives with breast cancer increases her risk fivefold.

Genetic predisposition: In a few cases, breast cancer is the direct result of a genetic mutation. If a relative's breast cancer developed before menopause, if it affected both breasts, or if she had ovarian as well as breast cancer, there's an increased likelihood that the cancer results from a genetic mutation such as the BRCA1 or BRCA2 mutation inherited from either parent, or from the interaction of other genes.

Talk with your clinician if you think you may be at risk. There is genetic testing available.

Menstrual periods/hormone exposure: Although we do not completely understand the precise roles that estrogen and progesterone play in a woman's breast cancer risk, the number of menstrual cycles she has during her lifetime appears to be related to her risk. Estrogen and progesterone are produced during the menstrual cycle—having menstrual cycles for more than forty years lengthens the cumulative exposure of breast cells to hormonal stimulation. For that reason, a woman's age at menarche (when she starts menstruating) and her age at menopause (when menstruation stops) are important in determining her risk. If menarche was early (age 12 or before) and menopause was late (after age 50) she has a slightly increased chance of developing breast cancer. This risk also exists if a woman has had no children or had her first child after age 30.

Previous breast cancer: Women who have cancer in one breast have about a 1 percent greater chance per year of developing a new, second cancer in the other breast or in the treated breast.

What you can do to reduce risk: Lifestyle factors

Although you can't control risk factors such as your gender, age, or family history, you can make some general lifestyle choices to help reduce your risk of breast cancer—and other cancers.

Alcohol: A moderate link exists between alcohol use and breast cancer. Wine, beer, and hard liquor can elevate the amount of estrogen in the blood, and anything that increases long-term exposure to estrogen can increase breast cancer risk. According to studies, having one drink a day or more appears to modestly increase breast cancer risk. The American Cancer Society's Cancer Prevention Study II evaluated the alcohol use of 490,000 middle-aged men and women over nine

Chances of Developing Breast Cancer

We often hear that one in eight women will get breast cancer. These are *lifetime* figures. Here are averages depending on age.

Age	All Women
By age 25	1 in 19,608
By age 30	1 in 2,525
By age 35	1 in 622
By age 40	1 in 217
By age 45	1 in 93
By age 50	1 in 50
By age 55	1 in 33
By age 60	1 in 24
By age 65	1 in 17
By age 70	1 in 14
By age 74	1 in 11
By age 80	1 in 10
By age 85	1 in 9
Ever	1 in 8

Note: Women with genetic predisposition for breast cancer have increased risks at earlier ages.

Source: NCI Surveillance Program and the Breast Cancer Linkage Consortium Guidelines.

years and found a 30 percent increase in breast cancer deaths among women who had at least one drink daily compared to women who didn't drink. Reducing alcohol consumption is one way to lower breast cancer risk.

Weight: The influence of weight on your breast cancer risk depends on several factors, including your age and whether you take hormone replacement therapy. But in general, avoiding weight gain during your adult years can help reduce breast cancer risk. The Nurses' Health

Study examined the association between weight and breast cancer risk and found that weight gain was linked to an increase in breast cancer risk for all postmenopausal women. Those women who had gained more than forty-five pounds since age eighteen had a small increase in risk of developing breast cancer. The more weight gained, the higher the risk.

Early detection of breast cancer

The earlier a breast cancer is found the better your chances for successful treatment. Early stages of breast cancer commonly do not produce symptoms, so it's vital to have mammograms and clinical breast exams according to schedule.

Breast self-exam: For more than thirty years, breast self-examination (BSE) has had a central role in breast cancer detection. This has helped make women more aware of changes in their breasts. However, during BSE women often detect lumps that are not cancer. This can lead to anxiety and sometimes unnecessary tests. Often changes in breast tissue are noticed at other times (for example: taking a shower or exercising). While it's important to notice and report any

Reducing Your Risk for Breast Cancer

- Eat a balanced diet high in fruits and vegetables.
- Reduce/limit consumption of alcohol.
- If you are taking or considering taking hormone therapy, ask your doctor to help evaluate your risk level. We know that hormone therapy is associated with an increased risk of breast cancer.
- Avoid gaining weight, particularly if you are postmenopausal.
- Talk to your doctor about regular screening.
- Exercise.

lumps in your breasts, because of its imprecise nature, there are changing opinions about the exact role of monthly BSE.

Some studies show that breast self-exam does not significantly help reduce the death rate from breast cancer. As mammography has become more popular, it has become the tool of choice. Nevertheless, by checking your breasts about the same day every month (seven days after your period starts), you are likely to notice changes that should be brought to your clinician's attention. However, remember that lumps, while important to make note of, are not automatically a reason to panic. Also remember that BSE is imprecise and should be used only to help detect *change,* not as a substitute for additional screening.

Clinical breast exam: Because about 10 percent of breast cancers are not found by mammography, clinical breast exams can be an important part of your health care. Some organizations recommend them every three years, others annually. It's a good time to ask your doctor questions about any changes you may have noticed. But like breast self-exam, it is not precise and should not replace regular mammograms.

Mammography: Mammography uses very low levels of radiation to X-ray the breast, and can find 90 percent of breast cancers. Right now, it's the most effective technique for finding early breast cancers. Mammography makes it possible to see tiny cancers before they can be felt as lumps. The masses that show up on a mammogram may be benign or malignant.

More than 75 percent of biopsies of suspicious tissue turn out to be benign. Since the 1980s, image quality has improved dramatically and the amount of radiation used has dropped. Accreditation standards that went into effect in 1999 closely regulate film quality, testing procedures, and training for technologists and radiologists. Most experts believe that mammography has contributed to the decline in breast cancer deaths since the 1990s. Other breast imaging technologies are in development and may someday become as common as mammography is today. These include digital imaging and even 3-D imaging. Both help make abnormalities more visible.

Breast cancer screening

Several authoritative organizations have published recommendations about the most effective ways to look for early signs of breast cancer in apparently healthy women. Two of the most widely regarded come from the U.S. Preventive Services Task Force (USPSTF)—a panel of health care experts who regularly evaluate data on disease and prevention—and the American Cancer Society (ACS). The two guidelines do not entirely agree.

The table on pages 248–249 summarizes the range of recommendations for women at average risk for breast cancer. Women at increased risk should talk with their doctors about the appropriate screening plan for them (which may include earlier screening and additional breast imaging technologies, such as breast MRI).

Treating and preventing breast cancer

If you are at high risk for breast cancer due to a family history or other risk factors, be sure to talk with your doctor about the right screening schedule and tests for you. Selective estrogen receptor modulators (for example, tamoxifen) offer some protection against breast cancer and may be appropriate for some women.

Selective estrogen receptor modulators (SERMs) and breast cancer: The FDA approved tamoxifen for breast cancer *prevention* in 1998, after the Breast Cancer Prevention Trial showed that women at high risk who took tamoxifen for five years had a 49 percent lower rate of the disease than women who were not on the drug. Raloxifene is approved only for preventing and treating osteoporosis, but it, too, shows promise in preventing breast cancer.

2003 Recommendation	Discussion
Mammography	
Starting at age forty, screening mammogram every one to two years	Research data have gone back and forth on the benefits of screening mammography. However, the most recent clinical trial results and meta analyses (studies that analyze the combined data from several studies) continue to show that mammography screening reduces the number of deaths due to breast cancer.
Clinical Breast Exams	
The ACS recommends that women ages twenty to thirty-nine have a breast exam by their clinician every three years; yearly clinical breast exams are recommended for women over forty.	Breast exam by a physician is another valuable screening tool, along with mammography. Women can take this opportunity to talk with their clinicians about specific concerns regarding breast health and breast cancer risk.
USPSTF judges the evidence as insufficient to recommend for or against clinical breast exam.	The risk of clinical breast exam is that it often detects "lumps" that turn out not to be cancer. This causes anxiety and additional testing that can involve radiation exposure, and the pain of a biopsy.
Breast Self-Exam	
It is important that a woman report any breast changes to her doctor promptly.	Some recent research suggests that breast self-exam does not significantly help reduce the death rate

The ACS no longer considers formal monthly breast exams an essential part of protecting breast health.

Neither the ACS nor the USPSTF actively discourages breast self-exam.

from breast cancer. One possible explanation is that as mammography screening has improved and become more common, breast self-exam has become less important.

This isn't to say that women shouldn't keep an eye out for breast changes. However, often lumps are detected not during a formal breast self-exam, but rather during other activities, for example, while showering, getting dressed, or during lovemaking. The key point of this change in the ACS guidelines is that formal monthly breast self-exams are not the only way for women to identify breast changes.

However, breast self-exam is one way for women to become familiar with what is normal for them and to identify changes. Any breast changes should be discussed with a clinician.

As with clinical breast exam, the risk of self breast exam is that it often detects "lumps" that turn out not to be cancer, causing anxiety and additional testing.

In 2002, following a three-year review of published research on tamoxifen and raloxifene, the U.S. Preventive Services Task Force issued guidelines about the use of these medications for breast cancer prevention. It recommends *against* the routine use of tamoxifen and raloxifene to prevent breast cancer in women at low or average risk. Yet it also says that a woman at high risk may benefit from such drugs. Whether she should take them depends on her health profile and personal preferences. A woman considering tamoxifen should talk with her clinician about the drug's potential side effects, which include blood clots in the legs or lungs, hot flashes, and increases in the risk of endometrial cancer, stroke, and possibly cataracts.

Memory and the Brain

All other things we study as neuroscientists are objective, public measurements of the organ we call the brain. The mind, even though it's produced by the brain and closely linked to it, is accessible only to its owner.

—DR. ANTONIO DAMASIO, NEUROLOGIST

If you've heard reports that lowered estrogen levels are linked to Alzheimer's disease (AD) and you've begun the process of self-diagnosis, you're not alone. Many women are a bit baffled and disconcerted by the suggestion that menopause affects memory. However, as we've outlined in Chapter 2, issues of memory apply to both men and women and are far too complex to be explained by gender specific hormones.

Alzheimer's disease isn't just trouble remembering. It is a degenerative brain disease characterized by continual loss of nerve cells in areas of the brain crucial to memory and other mental functions. Women appear to suffer Alzheimer's disease at a somewhat higher rate than men do. It's not at all clear, though, that the reason has to do with physical changes after menopause. One in ten people over the age of sixty-five and nearly half of those over age eighty-five have Alzheimer's disease. There are many confusing aspects of research on

Alzheimer's. Many of the studies are either done on animals or are observational studies, which as we've seen, have limitations. Data from a number of studies suggest that estrogen has beneficial effects on brain neurons and may improve learning and memory. Some observational studies in women suggest that estrogen used for at least ten years might delay or prevent Alzheimer's disease. However, in women with established Alzheimer's disease, randomized clinical trials have shown that estrogen is not effective as a treatment. Furthermore, combined hormone therapy (estrogen and progesterone) may actually increase the risk of dementia.

In another surprising turn of events, the Women's Health Initiative Memory Study (WHIMS) revealed that combined hormone therapy actually increased the likelihood of developing what was termed "probable dementia." Dementia involves the deterioration of intellectual faculties like memory and other cognitive abilities. It can be difficult to diagnose and, in the case of WHIMS, required researchers to use a cognitive questionnaire and enlist family members of the participants. The study set out to determine whether estrogen supplementation (either estrogen alone or estrogen plus progestin) reduces the risk of dementia in healthy women. More than 4,500 women over the age of sixty-five took part. These women took either estrogen (Premarin), estrogen plus progestin (Prempro), or a placebo.

Though the estrogen/progestin arm of the WHI was called off early due to concerns about an increased risk for breast cancer, researchers were able to use the early data to better understand combined hormone therapy and memory. The data showed that the risk of probable dementia for women in the estrogen plus progestin group was twice that of women in the placebo group. What's more, the evidence of increased risk was noticed as early as one year after the study started. And the differences persisted over five years of follow-up.

The results were considered unexpected and in stark contrast to earlier studies on the effects of hormone therapy on Alzheimer's disease and dementia. However, it is important to note that while the increased *relative* risk was twofold, the *absolute* risk was relatively small—resulting in an additional 23 cases of dementia per 10,000 women per year. The early results of WHIMS are further evidence that hormone therapy should not be considered as a preventive treatment for memory problems. As of this writing, the estrogen-only arm of the Women's Health Initiative continues and is expected to provide additional information about the effects of supplementing estrogen only. There are also questions about the timing of hormone therapy. Does starting HT at a younger age make a difference? All the women in the study were age sixty-five or older. Despite some unknowns, in light of the increased risk of breast cancer and heart attack reported, the WHIMS estrogen plus progestin data reinforce the idea that the risks of long-term combined hormone therapy outweigh the benefits.

Mind/body and memory

For women at menopause, issues of memory and clarity of thinking cannot be separated from contributing psychological and social factors. Stress, sleep, and mood, as well as hormones, all play a role. Just as there are things you can do to preserve your health, there are things you can do to protect your memory. What's great about these strategies is that many of them are good for your overall health.

Get a good night's sleep: People who don't sleep well at night tend to be more forgetful than people who sleep soundly. Try to shoot for a minimum of six hours a night.

Use your mind/body skills: Months and months of insomnia were the most compelling reason for Karen to join our program. She had begun waking up at three or four in the morning feeling warm and uncomfortable, with racing thoughts and heart palpitations. Her inability to get back to sleep triggered anxiety and fear about "never being able to sleep restfully again." Those thoughts worsened the insomnia.

Karen recalled sitting at her dining room table trying to write checks, but feeling as though she just couldn't do this task that she had done so many times. "I had always prided myself on having a good, sharp memory. All of a sudden it felt like things were out of focus and it was hard to concentrate. It was hard to move my mind from one thing to another and juggling things became very stressful. It was scary actually . . . I felt like my brain wasn't working properly and that generated a tremendous amount of mental stress."

For Karen, mind/body techniques were extremely helpful. Developing a regular relaxation response practice helped her to quiet her mind and alleviate much of the mental stress she felt. This, in turn, improved her sleep. "The breathing and relaxation techniques calmed my body, but also my mind. It slowed my thinking, I felt calmer, my mind was quieter so I could focus better." Mindfulness is another skill she, and others, find extremely helpful. "Mindfulness counteracted my sense of not being able to focus. It slows you down and makes you focus on one thing . . . staying in the moment. It took a few weeks, but I started to feel better and eventually it all went away."

Here are some ways many of our patients quiet their minds and get a more restful night's sleep:

- Develop a regular practice of eliciting the RR.
- Practice mindfulness: Do one thing at a time, and do it with your full mental and sensory attention.
- Practice self-nurture: When you feel rested, renewed, and energized you will be better able to focus/concentrate.
- Watch your thoughts: Reframe those that increase worry, anxiety, and stress and exacerbate insomnia.

Exercise: People who stay mentally sharp in their seventies and eighties also tend to get regular vigorous exercise. First of all, it's good for the lungs, and people whose memories and mental acuity remain strong in old age characteristically have good lung function, which is essential to delivering oxygen-rich blood to the brain. Second, exercise helps reduce the risk for diabetes and hypertension, illnesses that can be contributors to memory loss. And finally, animal research has shown that exercise increases the level of neurotrophins, substances that nourish brain cells and help protect them against damage from stroke and other causes.

"Exercise" the brain: Over time, people who don't challenge their minds have a greater degree of memory decline than do those who stay mentally active. Learn something new every day. Develop a lifelong habit of learning and challenging yourself mentally by doing things like reading, playing chess, doing crossword puzzles, or acquiring new skills. This mental activity is thought to help keep the brain in shape. So keep your brain busy!

Eat a healthy diet: A diet rich in antioxidants helps to neutralize free radicals, which can contribute to the aging of cells throughout the body, including the brain.

A Neuron Born Every Day

It was once accepted theory that our brain cells (neurons) couldn't regenerate. Scientists used to believe that we were born with a certain number of neurons, and that once these brain cells died, they were gone forever. This, combined with the fact that we lose about 10,000 brain cells a day didn't make a pretty cognitive picture for our later years.

Today, biologists have discovered that, at least in monkeys, thousands of neurons are born in the cerebral cortex each day. In 1998, researchers found that a group of brain cancer patients had sprouted new brain cells in the part of the brain called the hippocampus. These are encouraging findings.

Protecting your memory

The effort to preserve memory as we age is a prime area of research. But reports about research should not be taken out of context. Discuss any concerns with your clinician. Many conditions can trigger memory loss. So can some medications. If you suspect your memory lapses are not normal, a knowledgeable clinician is your best resource for evaluation and for the most up-to-date information in this rapidly evolving field.

Alzheimer's disease prevention: As mentioned, Women's Health Initiative data show combined hormone therapy (estrogen plus progestin) is found to increase the risk of probable dementia in women over the age of 65. So, hormone therapy should not be used to protect against Alzheimer's disease. Although an in-depth discussion of treatment options for Alzheimer's is beyond the scope of this book, there is a class of drugs approved for treating this disease. They're called acetylcholinesterase inhibitors (or AchE inhibitors), for example, donepezil (Aricept). Research on prevention and treatment continues, and progress is being made. For example, in October 2003, the FDA approved the drug memantine (Namenda). It is used for the treatment of moderate to severe Alzheimer's disease and is thought to work by blocking the action of the chemical glutamate. Several other medications under investigation look promising for prevention. These include other AchE inhibitors, anti-inflammatory agents, and antioxidants.

"Memory" supplements: Many "nutritional supplements" are marketed as effective alternative "therapies" for improving memory and many of our patients ask about these. Many have little or no solid evidence to support their use and limited data on effectiveness or safety. One of the most common is ginkgo biloba. A few studies have found a benefit from this herb, but others have not. So, additional research is needed to support the use of this supplement for Alzheimer's disease. If you take any blood-thinning medications (warfarin, aspirin, ibuprofen, and others), talk with your clinician before taking ginkgo biloba. There have been reports of some bleeding within the brain when used with such medications. And it should definitely not be used prior to surgery.

Achieving Optimal Health

By now, you've probably recognized how your lifestyle affects all aspects of your health. Think about the connections. If you don't take care of your body, you may be vulnerable to heart disease. Our cardiovascular system brings blood to our brains; thus lack of exercise and a poor diet might not only affect our hearts, but our brains as well. Watching for these connections may help motivate you to be good to your body.

From the brain to the bones, there are many ways to optimize your health. We suggest a combination of healthy lifestyle behaviors, the regular practice of the relaxation response, stress management techniques, and a willingness to work with your clinician to seek tested forms of preventative medicine. This means staying current on health screenings even if you think you're not at risk. In addition to monitoring your own health, keep track of research. New studies will teach us more about memory, diet, heart disease, osteoporosis, menopausal symptom relief, and a host of other issues pertinent to women. For more information about the latest studies, the following websites are helpful: The National Institutes of Health (www.nih.gov) and the North American Menopause Society (www.menopause.org). Discussing questions with your clinician will help you sort out how results apply to you.

CHAPTER 10

The Power of Your Mind

We are what we think.
All that we are,
Arises with our thoughts.
With our thoughts
We make our world.

—THE BUDDHA

A sk a dozen women about menopause and you're likely to get a dozen different answers. Even when symptoms are equally present, perceptions and attitudes can vary greatly. Gayle's view of menopause has been positive. She does not miss having monthly cycles, and in her professional life she's enjoying a newfound sense of acceptance and respect because of her age. "I can walk into meetings and sell ideas so easily," she exclaims. As a younger woman, she hadn't felt this ability to command respect. Despite dealing with hot flashes, Gayle feels empowered and ready for a challenge.

Linda's attitude has been different. "I had a terrible fear of menopause. I picked up a lot of negative information from the media. There were TV ads for medication to 'help' women with menopause. I got the idea that I'd look terrible, I'd gain weight, and so on." Fortunately, despite the power of her perceptions, Linda's fears were not realized. After participating in our program, where she learned to "restructure" her negative thought patterns, she no longer fears the transition, nor is she focused on worries about gaining weight or a change in appearance. Instead of falling victim to negative attitudes, she armed herself with information, learned to control symptoms, and challenged perceptions that were not serving her.

There are many perceptions in life that do not serve us. In this chapter, we give you the "cognitive tools" to recognize these thought patterns, reduce stress, and potentially transform your midlife experience. The idea is to create the life you want one thought at a time. After all, you are the maker of your world. We suggest making the best one possible!

Cultural Attitudes and Menopause

Attitudes are a powerful force. The bottom line: If we expect the worst, we just may get it! And attitudes about menopause, both good and bad, abound.

In Australia today, for most women, menopause signals wellness. In India the word menopause is translated as "the age of despair." In Greece it is viewed in more positive terms, signifying a "ridding the body of harmful vapors." In the Middle East it carries a spiritual meaning; it is considered an "age of pilgrimage."

How do cultural perceptions affect a woman's experience of menopause? While we cannot say for sure, it is interesting to note that in Japan, where age is respected, women report few problems. Overall, in cultures in which aging is given elevated status or in which menopause is viewed as a normal, healthy stage of the life cycle, women report menopause as being less problematic.

In the United States, where youth and sexual attractiveness are highly valued and emphasized, menopause and aging have traditionally been viewed with apprehension rather than respect. In the 1700s, words like "catastrophic attack" were used to describe it. Over the last century, terms like "ovarian failure" have contributed to the "medicalization" of menopause, by encouraging society to view it as a deficiency disease rather than a natural transition.

Fortunately, these attitudes are changing as women are learning to ignore and rebuke old stereotypes about menopause. As Dr. Susan Love puts it, "The menopausal ovary is neither failing nor useless. It is simply beginning to shift from its reproductive to its maintenance function. It's doing in midlife exactly what many people do, it's changing careers."

The Power of Perception

Things do not change; we change.

—HENRY DAVID THOREAU

If you've ever looked through a prism, you have watched light bend into many brilliant directions. Our perceptions work in much the same way. As we gather information from the world around us, we each put our individual "spin" on reality. We shape our perceptions based on our beliefs, background, and biological wiring. Sometimes these perceptions serve us well. Other times they can be a true barrier to happiness, creating "distorted" attitudes and beliefs. Thus, they color the way we view life.

The beauty of perceptions is that they *can* change! We create them and we have the power to reshape them. We can create perceptions that illuminate rather than darken our outlook. But it may take some work. Our underlying beliefs and attitudes have been forged over a lifetime—influenced, in part, by our culture, family, and friends. And the thoughts they generate have become automatic.

Negative Automatic Thoughts

Kate's day would often begin with a look in the mirror and self-criticism. "I look horrible," she would think, despite the fact that she was an attractive and successful businesswoman. "I'll *never* get everything done today," she would mumble to herself. Not surprisingly, she would go on to have a rough day.

Negative automatic thoughts are not something relegated to the years around menopause. Many of us have grown up with self-negating voices playing over and over in our heads like tape recorders. You may recall episodes as a teenager with friends where you would bemoan your own appearance and they would build you up again. As adults, we all know people like Kate, who constantly tell themselves they "won't succeed," they're "too fat," or they "don't look good," when you can clearly see that they've got nothing to worry about.

We generate automatic thoughts all day long. Our self-talk is constant and involves self-coaching, advising, criticizing, wishing, ruminating, and the like. These "tapes" play over and over again about the events in our lives, relationships, and interactions. If you were to examine the kinds of thoughts you generate during the course of a day, probably 90 percent of them would be negative, and of those, 90 percent are probably not true. Theorists, such as the psychologist Albert Ellis, have shown they tend to be knee-jerk reactions, based on our own perceptions. But like light filtering through a prism, our perceptions can be distorted.

Once you know what to watch for, negative automatic thoughts are easy to identify. The following words are usually red flags:

- Always
- Must
- Never

- Ought
- Should

Automatic thoughts sound like this:

"Oh no!"
"Why me?"
"I can't stand this!"
"I'm not good enough!"
"Nothing will ever change."
"This always happens to me."
"I'll never get everything done."
"How can I be so stupid?"
"I should have done better."
"It's all downhill from here."

The Negative Stress Cycle

Negative automatic thoughts can have a "domino effect," triggering negative emotions and affecting our health. Here's an example of how this works:

A woman is waiting for her doctor's appointment. She begins to wonder why she always has to wait. "I can't stand this," she mutters. "I'll never get out of here." "He always does this to me," she frets. As the minutes tick by, her thoughts turn to:

"I'm going to be late to my next appointment."
"My time means nothing to him."
"I'm going to find another doctor."
"He should know we're out here waiting."

These thoughts in turn affect her mood. She starts getting anxious, angry, impatient, and irritated that her time is being wasted. These begin to affect her behavior. Maybe she starts chewing her fingernails. Perhaps she begins pacing the waiting room or harassing the receptionist. These behaviors affect her physical well-being. By the time she is put into an exam room, where her blood pressure is taken, it is high. Now the worry is refocused. She begins to think new stressful thoughts:

"Oh no, now I have high blood pressure."
"What if I have to take medication?"
"What if I have a stroke like my mother did?"

The cycle continues.

Why are our thoughts so powerful? Imaging studies of the brain have shown that the very same area of the brain lights up whether you *look* at an object, such as a house or the letter A, or simply *imagine* that object. The woman at the doctor's office, imagining different negative scenarios, was feeding into a negative stress cycle and her body reacted. Our brain does not distinguish between thoughts and fantasies (what we imagine or perceive as a threat to our well-being) and true danger. The same cascade of stress hormones is activated. And, as we have seen, repeatedly triggering this fight-or-flight response can significantly affect your health.

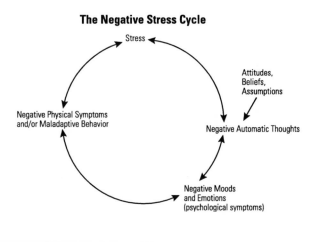

The Negative Stress Cycle

Stress

Attitudes,
Beliefs,
Assumptions

Negative Physical Symptoms
and/or Maladaptive Behavior

Negative Automatic Thoughts

Negative Moods
and Emotions
(psychological symptoms)

How do you stop the negative stress cycle? Like the "domino effect," if you change one of these factors, it results in a change in the others. So, you can break the cycle by intervening at any point. For example, if the woman at the doctor's office had been thinking about her new grandson or was focusing on an upcoming party, there's a good chance she would not have elicited emotions of anger. And there's even a chance her blood pressure may not have risen. Reading a book, chatting with the person sitting next to her, or listening to her RR tape are behaviors she might have used to break the cycle of escalating anger and frustration.

Cognitive Restructuring: Choosing Your Thoughts

So, if your "self-talk" is not serving you, *change* it! How do you get rid of automatic thoughts that just pop into your head? Like you would put out a fire! The "dousing" devices are awareness, logic, and reason.

Cognitive "restructuring," a central technique of cognitive therapy, pioneered by psychologist Aaron Beck, encourages us to see that stress does not always come from an outside event or situation. There is a great amount of stress that we generate on our own based on our thoughts. When we can recognize that some of our thoughts are "distorted," illogical, untrue, or not helping us, we can take giant strides toward changing our outlook on life. Several studies have shown that cognitive therapy is as effective as antidepressants in altering mood.

This is *not* about denying negative feelings or glossing over them. There are many events in our lives where it is appropriate to feel anxious, depressed, angry, and so on. This is about paying attention to our thoughts and changing those that are causing *unnecessary* stress.

Challenging negative automatic thoughts

Challenging and changing negative thoughts starts with asking yourself some basic questions:

- **Does this thought contribute to my stress?**
- **Is this a logical thought?**
- **Is thinking this way helpful to me?**
- **Is this thought true?**
- **Is this thought a "cognitive distortion"?**

Cognitive distortions

If your thinking contains one or more of the following characteristics, you may be suffering from what psychologist and author David Burns has called "cognitive distortions." Burns, a pioneer in cognitive restructuring techniques, compares the distortion effect to that of a strong pair of glasses that distorts our image of the world. See if you recognize your own thought patterns in the categories below:

All-or-nothing thinking: Situations are perceived as one way or the other. Everything is black or white; nothing is ever gray. If you can't remember something, you automatically assume you have Alzheimer's disease. If the lasagna you serve to guests one night is dry, you proclaim yourself a failure in the kitchen and vow never to cook again.

Generalization: When you experience a single negative event, you see it as part of a lifelong continuum. For instance, if a friend breaches a confidence, you feel as if you can never trust anyone again. If your spouse is late for dinner and forgets to call to let you know, you think things like "He always does this to me, I can't depend on him for anything."

Mental filter: You focus so much on the negative aspect of a situation that you fail to see anything positive in it. It's like adding a drop of black ink to a bowl of water. It colors everything. For example: you're at a party, having a wonderful time, when a friend says something like, "You look tired." You start dwelling on the comment and it ruins the entire evening.

Disqualifying the positive: When something good happens, you dismiss or devalue it. For instance, when someone pays you a compliment on a job well done, you say, "Anyone could have done it." Or you think to yourself, "They're just being nice." Although you might think you're being modest by deflecting praise, this type of cognitive distortion eventually makes you blind to anything positive in life. It's a way of turning positive events into negative ones.

Jumping to conclusions: This is automatically drawing negative conclusions even though there are no facts to support it. It involves predicting what others think or predicting the future. In some cases, you don't even try to do something because you are convinced you will fail. For example, you decide not to ask your boss if you can work from home two days a week because you "know" she'll say no, so what's the point?

Mind reading: You make assumptions about what someone else is thinking without verifying it. For example, you buy a birthday gift for a good friend. When you don't receive a thank-you note right away, you assume your friend hated the present. Or after giving a presentation at a business meeting, you ask for questions and there are none. You assume everyone hated the presentation and can't wait to get out of the room.

Fortune telling: Before you do something, you anticipate a negative outcome, assuming the worst is going to happen. This type of thinking is what is keeping many of us awake at three o'clock in the morning. "If I don't get enough sleep, I'll be a mess tomorrow."

Magnification (catastrophizing or awfulizing): You blow a negative event out of proportion, so that even a minor occurrence becomes a catastrophe. For example, you find out your refrigerator must be replaced, and you think, "That's it, I guess we're not going on vacation this year since all our money is going to go toward home repairs."

Minimalization: This is the exact opposite of magnification. You tend to dismiss or belittle anything good that happens, diminishing its importance. For instance, you receive a raise at work but you think, "What's the use? Uncle Sam will take half the money and what's left doesn't amount to much."

Emotional reasoning: You assume that your negative emotions reflect the way things really are: "I feel it, therefore it must be true." For example, you go to a conference where you feel inferior to other participants. Despite the fact that you are well prepared, you think to yourself: "I just don't fit in. I don't belong here, everyone here knows more than I do." Instead of reaping the benefits of stimulating conversation, you retreat and isolate yourself.

"Should" statements: You often find yourself saying or thinking: "I could have done it this way" or "I must do that." For example: "I should have gone to the gym today," or "I shouldn't have had that second dessert." The result is that you feel inadequate, pressured, anxious, resentful, and completely unmotivated. Should statements may bring to mind an image of an overbearing parent or teacher, wagging a finger at you. Albert Ellis called "should" statements a form of "musterbation."

Labeling and mislabeling: You define yourself, other people, and situations simplistically, on the basis of one negative event, rather than seeing complexity and variation. For instance, you skip going on your daily walk because you're tired, and then you think, "I'm such a lazy slob." Or you make a mistake and you think, "I'm such a loser."

Personalization: Somehow everything is your fault, even if you have nothing to do with it. For instance, your child does not behave well at a social event, and you think, "It's all my fault. I'm a lousy parent." Maybe one of your employees doesn't complete a task on time, and you think, "I should have done a better job motivating him."

Perfectionism: No matter how well you do something, it is never good enough unless it is perfect. You hold similarly high expectations for other people. For example, you feel you can only be happy if you are in the perfect relationship, your kids are all doing well, your house looks great, your career is successful, all your friends think you are great, *and* you are thin!

Challenging Cognitive Distortions

Before you can "restructure" an automatic negative thought, you must first put it to the test of logic. If it is untrue or illogical, there's a good chance it can be changed to better serve you. When an old knee injury ruled out running for Sonya, a cascade of negative thoughts filled her mind. She thought:

"My body's falling apart."
"I won't be able to run anymore."
"I'll never feel like myself again."
"I'm going to get fat and feel awful."
"I won't be physically attractive."
"My life is over."
"It's all downhill from here!"

We began to examine her thoughts. Were they helping her? No. Were they increasing her stress? Yes.

Needless to say her life was not over and the conclusions she had jumped to were not logical. Many of her thoughts fell into the above categories of "cognitive distortions" *(fortune telling, catastrophizing, jumping to conclusions)*. Once she became aware of these patterns she could begin the process of substituting healthier thoughts. For example, she agreed there were other exercise options she could sample, including yoga, swimming, or physical therapy, which would help strengthen her knee and keep her in shape. She was reminded that she was still perfectly healthy and full of vitality. Her restructured thoughts going forward became:

"I can explore other options to keep my body strong and healthy."
"I am a vibrant, attractive, and healthy woman."
"I can continue to be active and stay in shape."
"I can enjoy the challenge of trying a new exercise."
"I'll meet new people along the way."

By changing her thoughts, Sonya was able to change the way she felt. Feelings of depression, hopelessness, fear, and anxiety gave way to feelings of empowerment, self-efficacy and hope. The restructuring process helped transform her thoughts, her mood, and her behaviors. Sonya discovered she liked yoga. Restructuring her thoughts and softening her attitude about running was a process. She had to work at it. But, eventually, her knee got stronger, and in time, she was able to return to a more limited running regimen, which she combined with yoga. She ended up enjoying both.

Susan, a corporate executive, was in the middle of a large and important presentation. As she entered the critical phase of the presentation, she felt a hot flash coming on. Her immediate thoughts were not good:

"Oh no! Not now!"
"Everyone will know I'm going through menopause."

"I've lost control of my body."
"This will go on forever."
"This day is just a disaster!"
"I can't take it anymore."
"I can't live with these hot flashes."

Certainly thinking these thoughts could not only ruin a sense of confidence, but also throw off her entire presentation. The added stress served to exacerbate the hot flash. For Susan, the *catastrophizing, fortune telling,* and *mind reading* resulted in an increase in anxiety, less self-confidence, and feelings of embarrassment.

When we reexamined this scenario, we began to challenge the logic of her automatic thoughts. Despite her internal discomfort, Susan recalled that her hot flashes were not obvious to friends or family members. She also reminded herself that taking a deep breath and doing a "mini" could make the situation easier. After some discussion, she was able to come up with alternative, restructured thoughts that could be helpful if the situation came up again. These were:

"Take a deep breath and calm down."
"It may not be obvious and chances are no one will notice."
"Just go back to the presentation, it's going great."
"Ice water can help to cool me down."

After trying the "reframes" on several occasions, Susan found that limiting "runaway" thoughts decreased her stress, which was one of the triggers for her hot flashes. Armed with these reframes and her breathing techniques, she felt more in control and consequently less anxious. Her attitude about hot flashes changed to one of "I can handle it!"

Charlotte had just spent a week enjoying a fabulous and much needed vacation with her husband. The morning after arriving home, she got on the scale, weighed herself, and was dismayed to see she had gained five pounds. Happy thoughts of fun in the sun suddenly vanished, only to be replaced by the following self-critical thoughts:

"I'm out of control!"
"I did it again . . . I have no willpower."
"I'm so fat now!"
"I can't stand the way I look."
"What's happening to me!"
"I'll never fit into any of my clothes again."
"I shouldn't have gone."
"This is my husband's fault, he always wants to stop and eat!"

Charlotte, despite a wonderful week with her husband, was feeling regretful, angry with herself, out of control, powerless, unmotivated, unattractive, and miserable! She came to realize her thinking patterns often included *labeling, mental filtering, perfectionism, "should" statements,* and *catastrophizing.* A lot of women in our program identified with the scenario, so Charlotte got a lot of help in coming up with the following restructured thoughts:

"It's only five pounds!"
"I can lose the weight."
"I'm human!"
"I'll go to the gym tomorrow."
"I have a healthy diet."
"I'll wear my loose-fitting clothes this week."
"I had a wonderful trip eating and drinking with wild abandon doing *exactly* what I needed to do!"
"My husband and I really connected."

These kinds of restructured thoughts helped Charlotte to savor the memory and prolong the effects of her wonderful vacation. It moved her to feelings of self-acceptance (no one is perfect) with renewed enthusiasm for getting back to the gym and eating in a healthy way.

For Barbara, perimenopausal symptoms involved waking up at four o'clock in the morning and not being able to go back to sleep. At first she woke up feeling warm and uncomfortable, but over time, it was her racing mind that kept her up. Her negative thoughts at the time revolved around her fears of not getting enough sleep. They were:

"I won't be able to fall back to sleep."
"I'm going to be a wreck tomorrow."
"I'll never be able to function at work."
"Everyone else is fast asleep, what's wrong with me?"
"I'll never sleep restfully again."
"What if I need to start taking sleeping pills?"

Barbara's sleep was made worse by her thoughts. This is ultimately what prompted her to enroll in our program. Prolonged lack of sleep was affecting her moods, concentration, work, and really all aspects of her life. She felt out of control, anxious, scared, and hopeless. Barbara and the group worked together to try to come up with some reframes she could use at four in the morning (instead of *fortune telling, all-or-nothing thinking, catastrophizing,* and *labeling*). Her reframes became:

"I can listen to my RR tape, or do a mini."
"I always fall back to sleep sooner or later."
"I can usually manage on less sleep than I thought."
"If I'm up I can do some reading!"
"I have power over these racing thoughts!"
"This too shall pass."

These thoughts helped decrease her anxiety about sleep. She felt calmer about going to sleep, felt more equipped to cope with the four

A.M. wake up, and substituting these reframed thoughts helped her to stop worrying about it, which was one of the most strategic steps toward solving the problem.

Putting Reframing into Practice

Changing the way you think is a choice that will take time and practice. Initially writing down your thoughts will help you identify negative patterns. After jotting them down, challenge these thoughts. Do they fall into one of the cognitive distortions? Ask yourself, "Can I think of this in a different way?" Substitute more realistic and positive thoughts and beliefs, which will serve you better and promote health. They work best if they are short, positive, and just as powerful as the original negative automatic thoughts! Take a pencil and paper and try filling out a log based on the template below. This will help you identify and reframe cognitive distortions.

The Art of Coping

The well-known "serenity prayer," written by American theologian Reinhold Niebuhr, has been borrowed and adapted for many years.

Challenging Cognitive Distortions

Situation	Emotion(s)	Automatic Thoughts	Cognitive Distortions	Restructured Response	Resulting Emotion
Briefly describe the actual event leading to the unpleasant emotion.	Specify sad, anxious, angry, etc.	Write the automatic thought(s) that accompany the emotion(s).	Identify any distortion(s) present.	Write down a thought that serves you better.	Specify empowered, hopeful, etc.

Adapted from *Feeling Good: The New Mood Therapy*, by David D. Burns, M.D. (William Morrow, 1980).

Stop, Breathe, Reflect, and Choose

The Stop, Breathe, Reflect, and Choose approach is a great mind/body technique that can help you approach a variety of stress-inducing scenarios. Try it when you need to break a negative self-talk loop.

1. *Stop* yourself from responding automatically before your thoughts escalate into the worst possible scenario or you do something you might regret.
2. *Breathe.* Take a breath. Do a mini. This can elicit the physiology of the RR and divert your attention from the stressor and serve to redirect your focus.
3. *Reflect.* Focus your energy on the problem at hand and appraise the situation. Are you jumping to conclusions? What's really going on here? What alternatives do you have? By directing your thinking power toward alternatives and options, you'll pay less attention to those negative automatic thoughts.
4. *Choose.* Reframe thoughts that are not serving you. Choose the best way to deal with the situation at hand.

Essentially, its core words speak to everyone: ". . . grant me serenity to accept the things I cannot change, courage to change the things I can, and wisdom to know the difference . . ."

We cannot reframe all of life's scenarios. Some of our negative thoughts reflect "true" and "logical" difficult situations. When we are faced with such hurdles as a death, a failed relationship, divorce, the loss of a job, an illness, we must use a different coping strategy—one that involves problem solving and helps us move toward "acceptance." Our colleague Peg Baim, M.S., N.P., director of the Medical Symptom Reduction Program at the Mind/Body Medical Institute, has conceptualized a coping model that can be used for just about any situation. She emphasizes that the *essence* of coping is learning to make conscious choices and not simply reacting automatically. The *art* of coping is the balance between letting go and control.

273

The Coping Model

If a situation causes you to feel angry, stressed, anxious, or depressed:

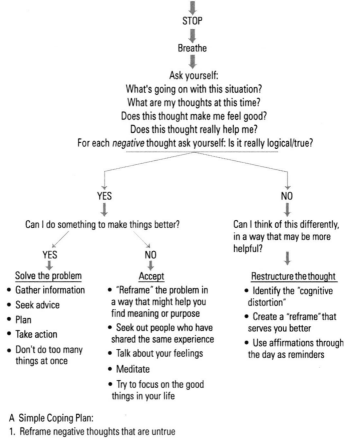

↓
STOP
↓
Breathe
↓
Ask yourself:
What's going on with this situation?
What are my thoughts at this time?
Does this thought make me feel good?
Does this thought really help me?
For each *negative* thought ask yourself: Is it really logical/true?

YES | **NO**

Can I do something to make things better? | Can I think of this differently, in a way that may be more helpful?

YES | **NO** |

Solve the problem
- Gather information
- Seek advice
- Plan
- Take action
- Don't do too many things at once

Accept
- "Reframe" the problem in a way that might help you find meaning or purpose
- Seek out people who have shared the same experience
- Talk about your feelings
- Meditate
- Try to focus on the good things in your life

Restructure the thought
- Identify the "cognitive distortion"
- Create a "reframe" that serves you better
- Use affirmations through the day as reminders

A Simple Coping Plan:
1. Reframe negative thoughts that are untrue
2. Problem-solve what you can control
3. Accept what's real by making meaning

Problem solving and acceptance

For Donna, perimenopause was difficult. She did not welcome the changes that accompanied the transition. An aspiring part-time actress, she lived an unconventional life. Surrounded by younger colleagues and friends, she had many issues around getting older. Because youth and beauty are highly valued in the acting world, she was stressed about the changes in her body. Her coping strategies involved taking up smoking again (after having quit for years) and eating, which served to create further anxiety. By the time she entered the program she was feeling old, unhappy with her weight, and her blood pressure was so high she was immediately started on medication. Donna's negative thoughts included:

"I'm getting old."
"My body's changing."
"My blood pressure can't be high . . . and now I have to take medication?"
"I hate this. I'll never feel myself again."
"My fellow actors will find out how old I really am."
"I won't get any more of the kinds of roles I want to get."
"I won't be physically attractive anymore."

The challenges for Donna were threefold:

1. Restructuring any thoughts that were distorted.
2. Problem solving her health issues.
3. Moving to acceptance about her age and life stage.

Donna did remarkably well in our program. She was diligent about eliciting the RR daily and began to exercise regularly. With the support of our nutritionist, she changed her diet. She then quit smoking. Three months after the program, she was able to discontinue her blood pressure medication. Donna's efforts are an excellent example of problem solving.

Accepting midlife changes was not easy for Donna. It was a process that required a little more "work." One of the exercises that helped, and that works for many of life's traumas, is borrowed from comic author Loretta LaRoche. It's called "Finding the Bless in this Mess." Take a piece of blank paper and for two minutes write down everything you feel blessed by in your life. This was a great exercise for Donna because it helped her refocus on all that she found wonderful and valued in her life.

Donna also reaped many benefits from the group support. There was much laughter and a few tears. Peer understanding and empathy, and the knowledge that others felt the same way, had a powerful effect in moving her toward a "reframe" of menopause and a change in her attitude about getting older. "Yes, this is a new stage of my life I can embrace," she thought. A couple of years after the group ended, Donna sent a note letting us know about an upcoming performance of a play in which she was appearing. After that, she was off for an extended jaunt in Europe, a new and exciting adventure. She was feeling anything but "old."

Pathways to Acceptance: Meaning Making

Ancient philosophers have long understood the healing power of acceptance. But the pathway may seem inaccessible at times. During these times, *meaning making* can help.

It had been nine years since Meg lost both her husband to cancer and her mother to heart disease. When the lump in her breast turned out to be cancer, she returned to a familiar place. In recounting the story of those difficult years, she became aware of the ways in which she had used meaning making as a way to help her cope and process her grief. She had diligently collected stories and photographs of her husband and mother to prepare for the two funerals. Through journaling, a symbolic tree planting, and the distribution of her husband's photography collection, she found tears and laughter in cherished memories.

Letters to family members and friends reestablished valued connections that helped with both losses. She corresponded with her husband's former students who came forth to reveal the most wonderful things about him. These sentiments became treasured gifts. She found meaning in working with his former colleagues and partook in the ceremonies when a wing of the university where he taught was dedicated in his memory. The paintings her mother had created became a source of strength and a reminder of her mother's gifts. In retracing the many ways in which both her mother and husband had touched the lives of others, she was able to reach acceptance and peace by focusing on the joy they had brought to the world around them.

Through the years, the process of searching for meaning had become familiar to Meg. As she faced her own cancer, she was, in some ways, prepared. She gathered information to help with her medical decisions, shared her journey with others, and searched for some inherent meaning in all of this tragedy in her life. Through her difficult times, she came to realize how many people were there for her, supporting her every step of the way. After radiation therapy, she pushed forward with a greater sense of purpose. She knew she had a very full and important life ahead of her. Fighter that she is, she's been cancer-free for three years.

Acceptance, in many cases, involves a different kind of "reframe," one that moves us to search for the inherent meaning in a tragic situation. To reach acceptance, we might ask ourselves: Is there some way I can grow and develop from this experience? What has this taught me? If we are faced with a serious illness like cancer, we might ask questions that seek insight: Has my life in some way been made richer from this experience? Can I look at this as being redirected to a new, perhaps more fulfilling path?

Social support, empathy, emotional expression, meditation, and prayer can all serve as pathways to meaning making. Techniques such as writing down thoughts in a journal can also be useful tools. Ultimately, if we can adopt the attitude that negative emotions and difficult times can be a catalyst for change, we can, in some cases, embrace times of emotional suffering. If we can appreciate that they can take us to a place of growth and greater understanding, we can, perhaps, consider them in a different light.

Healing Wisdoms

There are some emotions that can help spur us on in our search for acceptance. Two of these, *appreciation* and *gratitude,* can be vital to healing. Appreciation has been called the "gatekeeper of positive emotions." Even in the most difficult times, if we can embrace feelings of appreciation, gratitude, or thankfulness, we can open the door to a certain peace in our lives. This is the philosophy behind "Finding the Bless in this Mess." It can be as simple as being mindful of the small miracles and beauty around you: a child's smile, a mate's touch, an act of kindness. Cultivating an attitude of appreciation can move us toward emotions that better serve us.

Keeping a gratitude log

An appreciation journal or gratitude log can shift your mood. And it's simple to do. Each night write down at least three things that you appreciate about yourself or life. Hold these thoughts in your awareness until you feel a shift in your mood.

Lana's log entry: Lana had suffered through several miscarriages and was now facing early menopause. As she grieved the loss of never having a biological child, her husband, friends, and family all worried about her emotional health. Lana began seeing a therapist, but was having difficulty changing her focus of loss to anything else. She was unable to focus on any of the tapes we gave her. Nothing could seem to quiet the negative voices in her head. But when she learned about mindfulness, it triggered a change. She began to engage in mindful walks along the beach each morning, which she did religiously. At one session, we suggested she begin a gratitude log. She scoffed at the idea, but she was a very obliging person and reluctantly went about the task. Dutifully, she began keeping a very heartfelt journal. The following paraphrases her nightly writings:

I am thankful for:
The touch of my husband's hand
The smell of the salt ocean
The warmth I feel walking into a loving home
The strength and devotion of my husband
My extended family
Snuggling with my dogs
The support from friends in the group
My ability to nurture so many people in my life
My empathy

As Lana started holding her journal thoughts in her awareness, her outlook began to change. By the program's end, she felt more like herself. It was a gradual process requiring commitment, self-discipline, and hard work. She had learned to appreciate and focus on the things in life that she *had,* rather than dwelling on and longing for things she didn't have. And her husband was thankful for "getting his wife back."

Helen's log entry: Helen entered our program feeling depressed. Her relationship with her husband was difficult. He was controlling and critical. He was often not supportive of her endeavors. In fact he ridiculed her for joining our program. She had spent years internalizing the messages he sent. We suggested counseling and a consultation with a psychopharmacologist, but she had "been there, done that" and had already made up her mind to stay in the relationship for the sake of her children. She admitted that, critical nature aside, her husband was often very warm and loving. However, she felt somewhat trapped. At our urging she began to evaluate her commitment to herself. The idea of self-nurture was foreign to her. In fact, she admitted that she hadn't ever considered taking five minutes just for herself.

Embracing self-nurture and keeping an appreciation journal were turning points for her. At the end of every day, she was forced to find three things in her life she appreciated. She talked about her sons, her friends, the joy of discovering yoga, the relationships she was forging in our group, and her satisfaction with work. Her feelings about herself and her confidence improved. As she moved toward a more positive stance, and began to incorporate other skills she was learning in the program, she had more energy to set limits on her husband's comments and to create space for herself. It didn't move her to change anything in her situation, but her attitude shift created a very different life for her.

From Appreciation to Affirmation

In a sense, the ability to alter our lives for the better (to be happier) is just a simple attitude away. What we see and the meaning we attach to it is often a matter of choice or habit. The power to move beyond negative habits requires discipline and practice. One way to hold in our awareness the positive thoughts we have reframed or gleaned from our appreciation journals is to list those thoughts on index cards. Keep the cards with you and glance at them periodically during the day. These can become your *affirmations*. Some women hang them on their mirrors to view as they begin the day. Keep your affirmations short and simple. Deep philosophical statements rarely translate to our unconscious mind. For example, Helen, who was having difficulty with a controlling husband, carried a note to herself that read: "I can set healthy limits for myself." This simple reminder made her feel empowered whenever she glanced at it.

Here are some other simple affirmations generated by women in our groups:

I have the strength and skills to succeed.
I am more than my job.
My body may not be perfect, but parts of me are excellent.
I can handle this.
I can learn from my mistakes.
My best is good enough.
I embrace the challenge.

The Power of Contemplation

Another powerful tool we can use when we are "stuck" in negative emotions is *contemplation*. It can help move us to where we want to be, to feel how we want to feel, and can allow us to discover and move toward the life we want. Contemplation is a practice of meditation (see Chapter 3) that can serve to move us beyond negative emotions. During contemplation we can actually counter negative emotions by replacing them with positive ones. It is helpful, in practicing this, to identify and understand what is behind the negative emotions you are feeling. Usually you'll find they're driven by conditioned "underlying beliefs," which come from faulty emotional reasoning that has become habit. For example, let's say that you're feeling anxious. That is the "feeling." But what drives that feeling is the underlying belief that you are not safe or in control.

The following is a short list of some common negative emotions, and the underlying emotional reasoning which prompts them.

Feelings	Underlying Beliefs
Anger	Unfair
Anxiety	Not safe/not in control
Shame	You've done something wrong or you are wrong
Sadness	Loss
Guilt	Actions inconsistent from moral principles
Loneliness	Alone, and shouldn't be
Frustration	Unmet expectations
Inferiority	Compare yourself to others and fail to measure up
Jealousy	Wanting what other has

Source: Mind/Body Medical Institute. Adapted from *Feeling Good: The New Mood Therapy*, by David D. Burns, M.D. (William Morrow, 1980).

In embarking upon this type of meditation, first identify the emotion you want to move beyond. Once you have identified that negative emotion, consider the underlying belief. Now you can choose an *opposite* belief from the list of "healing beliefs" (page 283) to apply as an "antidote." Healing beliefs can transform your experience of a negative emotion into a more positive one. In a sense, the act of experiencing it in contemplation will be "healing." The healing beliefs we suggest emerged from a list of spiritual principles that come from the world's "wisdom traditions," among them Christianity, Judaism, Buddhism, Hinduism, Islam, and Sufism. There is no right or wrong belief. Pick one that resonates with you or that simply feels right for this particular meditation.

In the stillness of meditation, you can now "contemplate" the healing belief you have chosen. It is said that if your *intent* is to feel this way it will *become* your experience. For example, if you are try-

Virtues/Healing Beliefs

Abundance	Acceptance	Accountability	Appreciation
Aspiration	Awareness	Awe	Balance
Beauty	Beingness	Boundaries	Charity
Choice	Clarity	Commitment	Community
Compassion	Constancy	Cooperation	Courage
Creativity	Curiosity	Depth	Detachment
Determination	Devotion	Dignity	Discernment
Discipline	Discrimination	Economy	Enthusiasm
Equanimity	Eternity	Faith	Fearlessness
Fidelity	Flexibility	Forgiveness	Freedom
Friendship	Fulfillment	Generosity	Gentleness
Grace	Gratitude	Greatness	Growth
Harmony	Honesty	Honor	Hope
Hospitality	Humility	Individuality	Inspiration
Integrity	Intuition	Joy	Justice
Kindness	Kinship	Leadership	Loyalty
Love	Mastery	Newness	Nurturance
Oneness	Openness	Patience	Peace
Perfection	Perseverance	Positivity	Power
Presence	Process	Purity	Respect
Restraint	Serenity	Service	Silence
Sovereignty	Spontaneity	Stability	Stillness
Strength	Surrender	Tolerance	Transformation
Trust	Truth	Understanding	Vigilance
Vitality	Vulnerability	Will	Willingness
Wisdom	Worthiness		

Source: Compiled by Peg Baim, M.S., N.P.

ing to deal with feelings of shame (underlying belief: you've done something wrong), you might look at the list and decide to contemplate "forgiveness." Some people find it most effective to create an image of the healing belief, or imagine themselves filled with the emotion. For some, it is almost as if they "embody" the belief during their contemplation. Others find it easier to repeat the word or to use it in the following phrase:

> *Say to yourself:*   "I am filled with _____."
> *In our exmaple:*   "I am filled with *forgiveness.*"

If you sit in meditation for five to fifteen minutes contemplating a healing belief, you will feel a shift in your mood. In this example, once you move into "forgiveness" of self, it becomes more difficult to feel shame. In a sense the contemplation has transformed your experience of shame into self-forgiveness.

Tanya had been invited to present a paper at a prestigious conference in Chicago. Every time she sat down to organize her presentation she was paralyzed by her anxiety. "What if I make a mistake?" she thought. "I don't know enough to do this." "I can't do this!" We suggested that Tanya use contemplative meditation. Rather than falling into this negative thought cycle, she used contemplation to serve her better.

By referring to her list of "underlying beliefs," she reminded herself that her anxiety probably stemmed from underlying beliefs of not feeling safe (perhaps everyone would laugh at her) or in control (I can't do this). She needed an antidote that would return those feelings of control and safety. She perused the list of "Healing Beliefs." The word "power" jumped out at her as the right word to use. So she contemplated power in her meditation, working to transform her feeling of anxiety into a healthier one where she felt filled with strength. As she sat doing her deep breathing, her posture became straighter, and she sat taller. Every time she took a deep breath she felt more power. When she was done, she felt calm and empowered. She was able to continue preparing her talk. Her presentation was a success.

Contemplate what you want

Contemplation can serve as a wonderful emotional and spiritual boost. It opens us to new possibilities. It can move us toward acceptance and push us to reclaim what we want in our lives. By achieving inner stillness through meditation, it can also help us discover meaning, adopt new attitudes, receive answers, and develop insight. It can guide us when we need to move beyond negative emotions. It is not about logical thinking or analysis. Rather, it is in the experience of stillness that you become open to whatever happens. This is how answers come to those who contemplate.

A Contemplation Guide

If you think contemplation meditation is best left to Eastern monks who reside on mountaintops, you're wrong! Many of our colleagues who regularly practice contemplation rely on the following basic steps. Like any exercise, it may feel awkward at first, but keep trying.

Three Steps to Contemplation

1. **Find a positive focus:** For example, begin with a thought of appreciation or something that inspires you. This will move you to a positive mind state and allow you to more effectively maintain your focus. This makes it easier to quiet your mind.

2. **Find a repetitive focus:** Repeatedly focus on any combination of a word, phrase, or image until you get to quiet. (See Chapter 3.)

3. **Contemplation:** Once your mind becomes still you can harness the power of contemplation to replace a negative emotion with a healing belief. Or you can simply sit in the stillness of the meditation, pose a question, and wait for answers to come to you. It's a wonderful way to gain clarity and insight. You can ask, "What do I need to heal this [fill in emotion]?"

Remember: Your mind is a powerful tool—use it wisely!

What you think, you become
What you feel, you attract
What you imagine, you create

—THE BUDDHA

CHAPTER 11

Resiliency: Inner Strength

Let us not be enamored by the majestic oak,
For it is the bending branch of the tiny tree
that will withstand the greatest storm.

—ADAPTED PROVERB

We so often admire women who can weather any storm and still have the ability to smile. They forge on, hurdle barriers, and climb proverbial mountains to attain the best of what life has to offer. How do we follow in these footsteps? And can we look back on our lives and say, "I have lived the life I want!"

In many ways, embracing life is about finding the right pathway, making the journey, enjoying the view, and navigating the bumps. The last part may be key. Life has its share of rough times. Yet some people have a natural ability to "bounce" back from hardships, smoothing over difficulties with an uncanny ease. They don't let the little things get them down. They have characteristics that make them "stress hardy" and optimistic. This resilience is natural for some people. Biology, early life experiences, and family influences all likely play a role. But we are also finding that the characteristics of the "stress hardy" can be learned.

In the Footsteps of Stress-Hardy People

When psychologist Dr. Suzanne Kobasa conducted research at AT&T during the largest corporate reorganization in history, she found that people who were most resistant to stress shared three key characteristics, all beginning with the letter "C." They were strongly *committed* to (rather than alienated from) what they were doing at work and in their families and home life. They felt in *control* of their life (rather than helpless), so that they believed they could make choices that would influence the outcome of events. And they had an ability to view stressful events and change as a *challenge* or opportunity (rather than a threat).

During her study, Dr. Kobasa found that such "stress-hardy" people stayed healthy while others were more likely to become ill or be absent from work. To these three "C's" we have added a fourth, *closeness* or connection—that is, having people with whom to share. Substantial research has shown that personal relationships and other types of social support can provide a powerful buffer to stress.

Another approach to stress hardiness is offered by Dr. Barrie Greiff, a psychiatrist and business consultant who is also a former professor at the Harvard Business School. Greiff has identified what he terms the "five L's of success"—personal habits that correlate with health and happiness. They are:

Learn: People willing to learn also tend to welcome new experiences, rather than resist or worry about them.

Labor: People who work at something that they find satisfying and meaningful tend to be more positive than those who slog away at a job they despise.

Love: People who are in loving and reciprocal relationships—

with spouses, partners, or even friends—develop an inner strength that helps them be more positive.

Laugh: A sense of humor—being able to laugh at oneself or with others—helps people to view life in a more positive way.

Let go: People who are able to recognize times when they are not in control of something, and "let go" mentally, have more energy to direct at situations where they do have control.

How do we become more committed, more in control, and more able to view life as a challenge? How do we learn the "five L's of success"? It involves the many approaches we've outlined throughout the book. It also involves fostering emotional bonds, strengthening connections to others and to yourself.

Expressing Inner Emotions

When we laugh, love, learn, and commit, we express ourselves. The art of self-expression is a part of stress hardiness. Tapping our inner emotions helps us strengthen a commitment to ourselves. When we make the journey inward we can become more aware of our needs and understand what we are feeling. Learning effective ways to communicate what we feel not only helps strengthen our interpersonal connections, but the healing effects can be enormous. Releasing deep-seated emotions has been linked to improvements in both mental and physical health. Repressing emotions, on the other hand, has been linked to illness. As mind/body clinician Rachel Naomi Remen, M.D., has observed, "The only bad emotion is a stuck emotion."

Journaling: Carving a pathway for emotions

We have found journaling can be an epiphany of sorts for women, a time of realization and release. You may be familiar with keeping a diary, but the journaling we use in our programs involves a different process. It's a bit like burrowing into the depths of the soul and *allowing* the insight to come to you.

The week after we had assigned the journaling exercise to our group, as the women were sharing their experiences, Mary eagerly raised her hand and showed us a plastic bag containing a grayish powdery substance. She revealed that she had written for four days, as instructed, and then, on her own, set fire to the pages. The ashes were in the plastic bag. She stood up dramatically, walked to the trash can and let go of the bag. As it fell she stated, "I've been carrying this around for the last ten years and I'm ready to get rid of it!" We never did find out what she had written about, but a huge weight had been lifted from her shoulders.

Much of the work on the healing power of journaling has been done by James Pennebaker, Ph.D., a psychology professor at the University of Texas in Austin. In the late 1970s, Pennebaker began researching whether people who express their innermost thoughts and fears are healthier than people who do not. His research showed that writing about traumatic events could help people to deal with the negative emotions involved. People not only felt better, they *were* better, both physically and psychologically.

In one study, for instance, Pennebaker asked a group of student volunteers to write about superficial, nonemotional events for fifteen minutes a day, for four days. Another group wrote about traumatic incidents for the same amount of time. To further focus the research, the trauma group was divided into three subgroups: one wrote about only the facts of the event, another wrote only about the emotions it caused, and a third wrote about both facts and emotions. The researchers then determined the overall health of the student participants by comparing number of visits they made to the student health center in the months before and after the experiment. The students also filled out questionnaires about their mood several months after the experiment ended.

Students who wrote about traumatic events reported feeling happier after the exercise than students who wrote about trivial events. When the researchers analyzed the data further, they found that participants had to write about *both* facts and feelings in order to benefit. In the months following the experiment, those who wrote in detail about traumatic events, and explored the emotions involved in those events, made 50 percent fewer visits to the health center than other students. Those who wrote only about emotions, or only about factual details, visited the health clinic just as frequently as those who wrote about superficial topics.

In the decades since that first study, Pennebaker has taken the research even further. An analysis of blood samples from participants in some of these studies revealed that journaling increases levels of certain immune system cells, thereby bolstering the body's natural healing powers. Working with different colleagues, he has concluded that journaling improves health in a number of populations, including those with arthritis and chronic pain. Other researchers have corroborated these results more recently with similar findings in studies of patients with asthma and arthritis.

Picking up the healing pen: The journaling process is not hard, but there are a few guidelines to follow to get the most from your writing.

Sit for fifteen to twenty uninterrupted minutes and write about:

1. Any life crisis or difficult situation you have encountered.
2. Include both the facts and your feelings and emotions.
3. Repeat for three to four days in a row and stick to the original event or topic.

As you do this exercise keep the following in mind:

Pick an important topic: It can be a distressing event, a past trauma, or a situation that is nagging at you and you can't let go of.

Think about an experience that you've been mulling over, trying to resolve. Writing may help you to do so. Or think about something you would like to discuss, but are too embarrassed to talk about.

Write continuously: Pick a time when you won't be interrupted, because the goal is to write continuously for fifteen to twenty minutes, without taking your pen off the paper. It's helpful to use a timer. Don't worry about penmanship. In this way, you will access your innermost thoughts and will not give your "inner editor" a chance to stop you midstream.

Write for yourself: Although you may write your entry with someone in mind, and some people even write their entries in the form of letters to other people, keep the results private. Writing for yourself is the only way to ensure that you don't start shaping the narrative to avoid judgment from someone else.

Expect to feel something: As you do this exercise, you may initially feel worse. Negative emotions may surface. Fortunately these emotions usually begin to dissipate by the second or third day. By the fourth day, patients report their writing moves into a different realm—one of clarity, insight, acceptance, and forgiveness. It is almost as if the physical act of writing helps the brain process a traumatic event, and then move on. In the long term, most of our patients feel happier and at peace, an outcome borne out by Pennebaker's studies, which have found that the beneficial effects of journaling can last for several months.

Road Maps: Assessing Your Journey

Goal setting and taking stock of life events is another way to foster a commitment to self. Dr. Ann Webster, Harvard health psychologist, has worked to apply the concept of "road maps" for use in her cancer and HIV groups as a way to help patients make meaning of life's twists and turns. In our menopause program, this life review can be a powerful experience. Many women, looking back on difficulties and challenges in their lives, come to recognize and appreciate their own survival skills and resiliency. They remember mentors and teachers, people who have helped along the way. It is an exercise that allows women to reflect on where they've been (significant events, relationships, and accomplishments) and focus on what they'd like the next stage of their lives to look like.

Tricia, who had a very difficult childhood, used the exercise as a means of acceptance and enlightenment. She had come from a broken home in the inner city, married a drug addict, and raised two children as a single mother. Her map took shape as a winding road, with the early years filled with dark colors and ominous clouds reflective of the emptiness she felt during a lonely childhood, which included the death of her father. She portrayed the period when she met her husband with lightning bolts, creating the miracle of love but the pain of betrayal. The birth of her children was portrayed with bursting rays of sunlight. She considered her children the two biggest joys and accomplishments of her life. This entire middle section of her map was filled with pastel colors celebrating her joy in being a loving mother, getting out of a bad marriage, and making other healthy changes in her life. She had returned to school and her future road map was a portrayal of hope. Dancing figures, bright colors, and more light represented what she saw as endless possibilities. For the "gifts" in her life (her children), she added stars and blue skies. As she presented her road map to the group, her face was beaming.

Writing your road map: To create your own road map, think about the journey you have been on in life, and where you think you would like to go. Here are the physical steps; the imaginative part is up to you:

1. Find or buy some poster board.
2. Use the left-hand side of the poster board to depict the minor

and major events that have shaped your life, both positive and negative. If you do not want to work in a linear left-to-right fashion, you can designate a third of the poster board for past events.

3. Use the middle of the poster board (or another third of the total) to depict things you are currently doing—personally, professionally, spiritually, at work, etc.

4. Use the right-hand side (or final third) to describe your future goals.

Beyond these basic instructions, you can be as creative as you want. The following are some colorful road map variations we've seen in our groups:

The game board: Create a road map that resembles a board game. One patient came up with this idea, creating pleasant stops such as graduation from college, marriage, birth of a child, and birth of a grandchild. Interspersed with these were less happy stops, including the loss of a job and the death of a parent.

Photo collage: This is a popular way to construct a road map. Photos can be of family and friends, but they can also be pictures of habits you've quit (like cigarettes or junk food) or other ways of symbolically marking your journey.

Name the streets: Try adding a twist and naming "side streets" with names that are reflective of each period of your life. You'll be able to stand back and see the difference between, for example, the "Stress Expressway" and "Peace Lane."

Color coding: One woman placed colored stickers next to each significant event she recorded along a time line, running from left to right. The "good" events were assigned blue and purple stickers, while bad events were assigned orange and red. In this way, she could step back and see whether her life had been filled with mostly good things, or bad.

Building Community: Social Support

One of the true gifts women take from our programs is a sense of camaraderie. They feel it almost immediately. As they sit and share similar experiences, they realize they are not alone. For many, the responsibilities and demands of daily life have taken priority over creating time for connecting to female friends. They miss the friendships they had time to cultivate when they were young. And the discussions reflect this. They are dynamic, intimate, and range from symptoms, to sex, to new ways of viewing "the change." When you have a room full of women laughing about menopause, it can be a whole different experience.

The sharing is cathartic and the empathy healing. It can help women cope with symptoms and remain optimistic. Studies show that when peer support is combined with healthy lifestyle approaches, as we suggest, women reap long-term benefits that last even after participation in the program ends—including a boost in self-esteem and physical health. One of our patients recently admitted that she really missed a ritual the women in her group had created of meeting for coffee before each session began. These women had formed a cherished bond.

Healing and social support

The healing effects of social support were seen in a landmark study involving women with advanced breast cancer. In 1976, David Spiegel, a psychiatrist at Stanford University Medical School, organized what he thought would be a limited one-year research study to test a new kind of "supportive/expressive therapy." Spiegel was concerned about the emotional state of women whose tumors had metastasized. Their prognosis was grim. Spiegel believed that in addition to physical pain, these women also experienced an emotional isolation from family and friends. He hoped to break through that isolation with weekly support groups of women who shared not only the same diagnosis, but also the same fears, frustrations, and even small triumphs.

The women formed an almost instantaneous bond. Tears, laughter, and fear poured out as they revealed similar stories of well intentioned but clueless friends, loving but obtuse husbands, and terrified children. Spiegel's study compared women participating in the support group in addition to their standard medical treatment to a control group of women who continued medical treatment without a support group. After a year, he found the women in the support group were significantly less anxious, less depressed, and more confident that they could cope. There was a definite change for these women. And a decade later, after rechecking his data for another purpose, Spiegel found the women in the support group had lived twice as long as the women in the control group, an average of thirty-eight months versus nineteen months.

The data on social support and health are now overwhelming. In fact, loneliness and social isolation is comparable to smoking in its negative affects on health. During a six-year Swedish study, more than 17,000 men and women were followed. Those who reported being most lonely and isolated were nearly four times more likely to die prematurely than those with an adequate social network. This risk factor was independent of other risk factors such as age, smoking, sedentary lifestyle, and poor diet. In fact, nothing could explain the relationship between early death and social isolation. Similar studies have all come to the same conclusion.

Bonds with friends and family

Social support is a bit like an umbrella, sheltering us from the stresses of life. A good social network will offer emotional, physical, psychological, social, and spiritual aspects that work together. The people in your network may consist of family, friends, coworkers, and acquaintances. While your family can be a primary support system, it's good to have different types of support. For instance, having a group of great girlfriends is a gift that should be cherished. Women can provide immense coffers of support for each other. So make room for it. After all, comparing a night out with "the girls" to a family get-together is a bit like comparing apples and oranges. You just can't. Both offer emotional rewards and contribute to a more stable social network.

Sizing up your social support: Having a lot of family and friends does not always equate to a balanced support system. For instance, who can you count on to call at three o'clock in the morning if you really feel distressed? Are you usually the one "giving" in your relationships? How often do you receive the support you need? A good way of looking at the type of relationships you have is to begin to think about your social circle. We like to call it your "social atom." Like the nucleus of an atom, you are at the center, surrounded by friends, family, relatives, colleagues, and acquaintances. Similar to an atom and circulating electrons, there is an energy exchange between you and those around you. We have our patients fill out the Perceived Energy Exchange Evaluation. It helps to determine in which direction the energy is flowing. If it's all flowing out from the center (you), with very little flowing in, you may want to consider reconfiguring your social circle.

When you look at your "energy exchange," are you giving 90 percent to some people and getting back only 10 percent? Each relationship has its unique balance of give and take. For example, kids, pets, and work may require a lot of energy. But they give back in different ways. Quantifying and justifying percentages is not the goal of the exercise. Rather, use it to spot disproportionate exchanges. For

Perceived Energy Exchange Evaluation

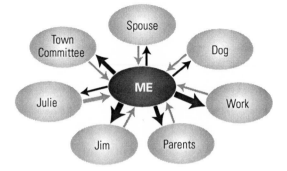

example, if work is taking over much of your life, yet it does not provide a sense of accomplishment or fulfillment, this may be an area to analyze. If you are "always" the source of support for a needy friend, but she's never there when you need her, it may be time to reconsider the friendship or add new friends to your circle. After considering your "energy exchange," try answering the following questions:

- For those in your life with whom you have a problem of energy exchange, can you make changes or problem solve?
- Are there people in your life whom you can really count on, but do not have regular contact with? Do you want to add them to your circle? Do you want to get in touch with them?
- Are there "toxic" people in your life? If so, can you set limits with them or limit the amount of time you spend together?
- What are your needs? Think about who can fulfill them. What's missing in your relationships? Where do you want to go from here?

One of our patients, Brenda, admits to having friends that can be very needy. Her response is to be helpful, but give herself emotional room when she needs it. "Instead of getting too involved, I listen to what they're telling me and pretend I'm watching a movie. I am far less drained if I can avoid adding their stress to my own." Brenda has successfully cultivated the skill we teach in RR of "nonjudgmental awareness," that is, being able to simply "observe" and "witness."

It may become clear that some people are able to provide emotional support, while others cannot. To find the support you need, you may need to reach out to new groups of people. Remember that the quality of our relationships is just as important as the quantity.

Setting boundaries

Learning to set limits and maintain boundaries is helpful in renegotiating "toxic" relationships and creating healthier ones. It is another essential part of self-nurture. (See Chapter 4.)

One of our patients, Fran, complained one day about the route her life was taking. Her youngest child had just gone off to college, and she had mixed feelings about that. She had barely begun to think about her own needs and the possibilities of new ventures when it became clear that there were other plans for her time. Her mother-in-law, who happened to live downstairs, had many physical and emotional needs. Her husband assumed that, now that the kids were gone, Fran would take on those responsibilities. After all, she had spent her life caring for others. Before she knew it, her life began to revolve around her mother-in-law's needs.

Fraught with a mixture of anger, resentment, and guilt, she felt paralyzed. She did not know how to say "no" to her husband or mother-in-law. With the support of the group, she was sent home with a few productive ways of communicating the word "no." After some negotiation, she convinced her husband to hire some part-time help. Fran began to set limits, to make time for her own needs, and to think about what she wanted for her future. Miraculously, the tension in the relationship with her husband improved and her mother-in-law was fine. For Fran, the results were like a weight being taken from her shoulders. "I feel much more energetic and joyful and interested in my life again, as I have made more space for myself and my needs." While saying "no" and asking for what we need can be difficult, we have found that with practice—and a few tips—it becomes easier.

Saying "no": For many of us, saying no brings up feelings of guilt, discomfort, anger, dishonesty, and rejection. It can clearly add stress to interpersonal relationships. One thing to remember: when you say no you are saying no to the request, you are *not* rejecting the person. Try experimenting with the following approaches. You can mix and match depending on the situation.

No #1: A simple "no" approach works best when a simple response is sufficient.
No #2: No, because _____. (*Give an honest explanation.*)
No #3: No, but how about _____? (*Offer a compromise.*)
No #4: No, but let me think about it and get back to you. This is often the easiest for "beginners" because it allows for time to think about your needs. Will this push me over the edge? Can I really take the time? Based on your needs, decide yes or no. Of course, it's important to follow up and get back to the requestor in a timely fashion.

If "no" is typically not part of your vocabulary, practice it! Ultimately, it's worth it.

The art of communicating

Talking is easy, talking well is a bit tougher—and good communication is a complex web with many layers. When we communicate effectively, it reduces stress, improves relationships, boosts self-esteem, and provides a hardy internal buffer. When we don't communicate effectively, it can have the opposite effect.

Four communication styles: There are four basic ways that people communicate: aggressive, assertive, passive, or passive-aggressive. Only one of these styles is productive. Understanding the differences is easiest if you can actually envision a conversation. Here's an example. Let's suppose you had a hard day at work and now you're at the store with your teenager, rushing to get him equipment and to a game. You race through the store, grab your items, and then make a beeline for the checkout counter, where many people are waiting.

A woman with a shopping cart full of items nudges her way in front of you, though you've been standing patiently. Which of the following statements comes closest to describing what you would do?

- *Option 1.* You poke the person on the shoulder and say, "Hey, what do you think you're doing? I've been standing here for a while. Go over to that other line or get behind me!"
- *Option 2.* You tap the person on the shoulder and say, "Excuse me, you may not realize that I was here first. You've got a lot of items in your cart. I'm in a big hurry. Please wait your turn."
- *Option 3.* You want to say something, but you don't. You just stand there and "awfulize" the situation, thinking, "People are so irresponsible. I'll never get my son to the game on time. This always happens to me."
- *Option 4.* You tap your foot loudly and exhale loudly with disgust. Maybe you even bump into the offending person. Or express loudly to the person behind you how inconsiderate *some* people are!

Now let's see what each option reveals about your communication style.

Style 1—Aggressive:

Someone who communicates aggressively is sending out a strong message to the other person, "I count, but you don't." Aggressive communicators always seem to be on the attack. The language used is threatening and often hostile. This only serves to escalate emotions and will rarely result in getting the reaction you want from the other person.

Style 2—Assertive:

An assertive communication sends out the message, "We both count." The language used is not emotional. It acknowledges and respects the other person's perspective, but also allows your own opinion to be heard. This kind of communication style can effectively strike a healthy balance in negotiating a satisfying outcome. The *assertive* communication style is most productive because it enables you to honestly express your feelings, opinions, and positions in a way that also is respectful of another person. It is a style that allows room for negotiation and choice.

Style 3—Passive:

In a passive communication you do and say nothing, even if a situation bothers you and you are seething inside! The message underlying a passive communication is, "You count, but I don't."

Style 4—Passive-aggressive:

The message being communicated here is, "I count, you don't count, but I'm not going to let you know it." Of all the communication styles this may be the least productive, because it is not an honest communication and leaves the other person guessing why you are doing something or why you are angry.

As you focus on what you say, also pay attention to how you say it. There are times when our body language can be a roadblock. Pay attention to your stance. Are your arms clenched? Are you unknowingly frowning? Your body language, facial expressions, eye contact, gestures, and actions may all convey as much, or more, than your words.

Expressing anger

Stacey began to notice that she would leave conversations irritated, even seething with anger. You wouldn't know it by the look on her face. She would retain a smile or appear unaffected. When she walked away it was another story. Stacey had long had a problem with hiding anger. When she did express it, it often surfaced in a passive-aggressive manner, and she was beginning to see the stressful toll it was taking on her. She relayed the following story to us in group: One cold, snowy morning she had shoveled snow from her walkway. That afternoon a young man, attempting to dig his car out, was inadvertently putting fresh piles of snow back on her walkway. Furious, she exclaimed, "I don't think you should be doing that." His response was to make a vile comment and continue on. Stacey said nothing and walked inside. She was much angrier than before. After about ten minutes, still not saying a word, she proceeded to vent her anger in silence by shoveling the snow back onto his car. She had worked herself into a frenzy, getting so upset she was red in the face. While it appeared she was getting back at him, it was actually Stacey who was suffering.

Learning about different communication styles and the "Stop, Breathe, Reflect, and Choose" approach to stressful situations resonated strongly with Stacey. Recalling the snow-shoveling incident, she has a new perspective: "I know now if I had stopped, observed what was happening, and asserted myself, I would not have gotten to that level of anger. What I needed to do was tell him he had no right to speak to me in that way." Stacey realized that making an assertive statement would have allowed her to maintain her own integrity while communicating a strong sentiment that she would not allow herself to be treated in that manner. By learning to express her anger in a healthier way, Stacey has been able to overcome old barriers of fear that had kept her anger bottled up.

A lot of women have a hard time expressing anger constructively. Some, like Stacey, have a fear of what others will think if they become angry. Cultural messages have made some women feel it is inappropriate to express anger. Other women fly off the handle if even slightly provoked. Bottled up or explosive anger is harmful to your health and relationships. However, if guided correctly, anger can be a powerful way of making your needs known. In the book *The Dance of Anger,* psychologist Harriet Lerner, Ph.D., makes an observation: "Anger is a signal, and one worth listening to. Our anger may be a message that we are being hurt, that our rights are being violated, that our needs or wants are not being adequately met, or simply that something is not right."

The following questions can help you develop a greater awareness of the nature of your anger:

1. It makes me angry when ____.
2. When I get angry, I'm afraid that ____.

The imagery-based RR described in the sidebar can be helpful in acknowledging, understanding, and learning how to manage anger in a more healthy way. It can be used for all types of emotional exploration.

Effective listening

Just as you would be mindful of a gorgeous day, be mindful in conversations. So often when we listen we do just the opposite. We are formulating responses and advice even before the other person is finished speaking.

Guided Meditation on Emotions

Allow yourself to be comfortable and relaxed, close your eyes, and imagine yourself walking across a small meadow—feel the breeze, sun, etc. Allow yourself to truly be in this experience, feeling all your senses. Journeying through the meadow often takes three to five minutes, during which you notice that the meadow is lightly ringed with trees. Soon you enter this forest and find yourself drawn to a hollow tree. As you stand before this tree, call out an emotion that you find burdensome and too often/easily experienced, one you wish would be less easily expressed or experienced (for example, fear, anger, anxiety, sadness, depression, betrayal, jealousy, guilt, loneliness, or hopelessness).

Observe this specific emotion mindfully as it emerges from the hollow tree. Without judgment, notice its size, color, shape, texture, any particular odor, and how you feel in its presence.

Next allow yourself to sit across from this emotion and honor it for protecting you. It likely presented itself to you when you were young and had little else to rely on. Even if it's an emotion you have significant trouble with now, still thank it for doing its best to protect and defend you in your youth.

Next begin to converse with the emotion, letting it know how you now feel and of your request for it to be less easily and often expressed. Listen to its wisdom. It will probably tell you why it persists and what it is you need to do for it to subside. Perhaps there's some arrangement or deal you want to make with it. Try asking the emotion to speak to you first before it lashes out next time. Listen for a reply, if there is one, and be there with it in the stillness, breathing together for a few more moments. After two to three minutes or so, say goodbye in any way that feels appropriate. As you prepare to leave, notice whether your emotion changed in any way (size, color, shape, smell, texture, etc.), and finally, decide what is best to do at this point. Do you want to take it with you, put it back in the tree, drape it over a rock in the sun or shade? Do whatever feels fitting.

For balance, flexibility, and direct positive influence, revisit the tree and ask that a more positive emotion emerge, one that you wish you would express more often and more easily. Proceed just as you had done with the negative emotion.

The following is a great exercise to try with a partner, whether an intimate mate or a good friend. It enhances communication and nurtures a sense of togetherness.

To begin, speak about a personal issue, feeling, or experience of significance to you. Without saying a word, your partner listens mindfully for five minutes, hanging on your every sentence. Now, switch roles. For five minutes listen intently to what your partner has to say. When we have the floor to speak freely without interruption, analysis, or argument, we feel like we're being heard.

Now try a variation on this exercise. During your speaking time each of you addresses the following questions:

- Something you like about your partner you have never told him/her
- Something you like about yourself you've never told him/her
- Something you like about your relationship you've never told him/her

Each of you should speak on the topics, uninterrupted, for a few minutes before giving over the floor to your partner, who then does the same. After you've both had a chance to talk uninterrupted and have been listened to with mindful attention, take five minutes to discuss what you've heard. Many women who try this with a partner are touched by the things that are said during these mindful moments.

"News and goods": The "news and goods" exercise, as the name implies, is a way of increasing mindful awareness of the positives in our everyday life. How often do you arrive home and begin by venting about the pitfalls of the day? "News and goods" is a simple antidote to creeping negativity in any relationship. Each person is asked about one thing that happened to him or her that day (or in the recent past) that made them feel good. It can be new and good or simply good. The exercise involves greeting your partner each night with the following question, "What new and good thing happened to you today?" After they explain theirs, talk about yours. "News and goods" can be something as simple as a funny conversation, getting change back from a vending machine, hearing from an old friend, a smile from a stranger on the street, making the light you always get stuck at on the way to work, or a compliment from your teenager. When you start a conversation this way, it can truly change the tone and mood of an entire evening. It engenders a sense of closeness and connection.

One woman admitted her nightly commute home with her husband had become mundane. Both would begin the drive venting about their days. This would lead to discussions about bills, refinancing the mortgage, or other lists of "things to do." When she tried the "news and goods" exercise, she noticed a marked difference. The first night her husband had to digest the question, then beamed, "I won the football pool." This simple comment resulted in the couple talking about where to celebrate, when to start taking dance classes, and hopes for a long-overdue vacation. They got home laughing.

"News and goods" can be helpful at any time of the day, in any situation. Patients who are teachers use it in their classrooms, others as an opener for family dinner conversations, or in staff meetings. The only thing you don't want to do is qualify it with a *"but."* For example, "I bought a new outfit for myself, but it cost so much money and I shouldn't run up my credit card." "News and goods" is a way of drawing on the positives of the day, and leaving the negatives behind.

Humor Replacement Therapy

One of the best prescriptions for life's ups and downs is available at any moment of the day. Laughter is good medicine and filling the prescription can be as simple as looking at the comics section of the newspaper or calling a friend.

Healing with humor

For thousands of years humans have acknowledged the healing power of humor. In the Bible it says, "A merry heart doeth good, like medicine." Today, science backs up this ancient wisdom with evidence that should make humor part of any good health plan. It turns out hearty laughter has the ability to reduce pain, create a mild state of euphoria, and boost the immune system. Research also suggests that people who use humor suffer less fatigue, tension, depression, and confusion in response to stress. Humor is even linked to pain reduction.

Humor and coping

You could be having a bad day. Hot flashes could be bothering you. You're late for an appointment. Your place is a mess. Nothing is going right. And in the midst of turmoil, if you force yourself to smile, you will feel better. Maybe just a little, but it's a start. Research shows that by changing our facial expressions we elicit corresponding emotions. Frowning can actually make us feel sad, while smiling can make us feel happier. And laughter is a smile, magnified.

When we laugh, we physically dampen the effects of stress. Laughing provides a timeout and has a way of automatically restructuring negative thoughts. It allows us to see a silver lining when a dark cloud rolls in. And it offers us respite from the stresses of life. Thus, it is a wonderful tool for coping. It's also a great tension breaker, reducing barriers between people and increasing a sense of connection. As Victor Borge once said, "Humor is the shortest distance between two people."

Your humor prescription

In addition to being health promoting, humor is *fun*! Yet, how often do we work it into our days? Think of it as a skill and practice. Here are some ways:

1. Make time for funny movies, plays, comedy shows, or cartoons. Even at times when you're most upset, these can brighten the picture and help break the stress cycle.
2. Set a mental channel for humor. Look around you (any room, anywhere) and find three things that make you smile. As Dr. Seuss said, "From there to here and here to there, funny things are everywhere."
3. Wear a smile whenever you can (as you get off the elevator, walking down an aisle, in a supermarket, driving in a car). Loretta LaRoche, who has been called the Erma Bombeck of stress reduction, calls this the "fake it till you make it" approach. A smile can change your attitude.
4. Do something nice when someone least expects it.
5. Get in touch with the child within . . . *giggle, twirl!*
6. Spend time with people who make you laugh.
7. Exaggerate. If you're having a bad day, then *have* one! Complain all day. Write a letter to your "higher power," unleashing your fury. Then answer it. Exaggeration is a natural way to reduce stress and anxiety because it helps us stand back and take a fresh look at the situation. If we can create a mental sitcom, overdramatizing anything and everything, and then laugh about it, we can't help but put the actual situation into a better context.
8. Create a *humor pot.* Mary Labuzienski, M.S., an exercise physiologist at one of our MBMI affiliates, has found a great way to motivate people in our programs to laugh out loud. She creates humor pots filled with hundreds of slips of paper, each containing a joke or a funny line. She calls them "Laugh Lines for Life's Little Wrinkles." Anytime you see a funny joke, a quote, or anything absurd, humorous, odd, inspiring, or in any way laughable—jot it down on a slip of paper and add it to your pot. Ask friends to contribute their lines. And

when you need it most—even when you don't—pick from the pot. Use it at home, work, class, parties, anywhere. If somebody else is in the room, pass it along. Laugh Lines for Life's Little Wrinkles can be a great way to stop, take a breath, and laugh.

Sample Laugh Lines

Sometimes I feel like a three-pound hen trying to lay a four-pound egg.
—Anonymous

I've been on a constant diet for the last two decades. I've lost a total of 789 pounds. By all accounts, I should be hanging from a charm bracelet.
—Erma Bombeck

I'm not afraid to die; I just don't want to be there when it happens.
—Woody Allen, *Without Feathers*

The chief cause of stress is reality.
—Lily Tomlin

I read this article. It said the typical symptoms of stress are eating too much, impulse buying, and driving too fast. Are they kidding? This is my idea of a great day!
—Monica Piper

Source: Compiled by Mary Labuzienski, M.S.

Characteristics of Happy People

Perceive the world in positive ways
Appreciate themselves
Believe in development and growth
Like other people, but don't compare themselves to others
Value the world at large
Live in satisfaction

Whether it's laughing, reaching out to loved ones, or tapping inner emotions, there are many ways to develop stress-hardiness. The approaches outlined in this chapter have helped many women overcome obstacles, improve their midlife experience, move toward happiness, and have fun in the process.

A sense of humor can help you overlook the unattractive, tolerate the unpleasant, cope with the unexpected, and smile through the unbearable.

— MASHE WALDOKS

CHAPTER 12

Putting It All Together

A journey of a thousand miles begins with the first step.

—LAO-TSU, CHINESE TAOIST PHILOSOPHER

When you look at a great painting, you're seeing thousands of brush strokes. Brought together, they become a work of art. Many important things we do in life are the result of a building process. The way we approach health and happiness is no different.

You now have a toolbox of skills and knowledge about health care decisions that can help you manage symptoms of menopause and stay healthy. But, like the brush strokes in a painting, the tools we offer are designed to work together. These techniques can dramatically change the way you feel. Mind/body approaches are not quick-fix solutions. They are meant to last you a lifetime and require practice and a commitment to "self."

Rachel recalls overcoming a few physical and mental barriers in the beginning as she worked to elicit the relaxation response (RR). Bothered by hot flashes mixed with anxiety, she initially had a hard time "quieting" her mind. Her "physical" barrier was a busy life that included two teenagers. Her "mental" barriers involved a lack of focus, due to racing thoughts about obligations. With some practice, she was able to overcome these barriers and allow the process to happen. Once she mastered it, she learned to calm anxiety, slow a racing heartbeat, and clear her mind with the RR in just twenty minutes. In her words, "It's like learning to ride a bike. It can take a lot of repeated tries before all of a sudden, you get it." Today, Rachel has regained the life she loves and continues to employ the full "toolbox" of skills she's learned.

The Mind/Body Approach

The mind and body are inextricably linked. As you go forward, remember the basic ways to tend to both:

Nourishing the mind: Nourishing the mind and spirit involves taking time for yourself. A daily meditation practice involving the RR yields both physiological and psychological benefits. But if you don't take the time, you won't reap the benefits. Practiced daily, the RR can help you become less reactive to the stressors of daily life. And you may begin to notice, as do many of our patients, that when you *don't* do it, you feel more bothered by symptoms and less able to "roll with the punches."

If you don't have twenty minutes for a meditation, take five. Five often stretches to ten. For Helen, a regular RR practice combined with "minis" have allowed her to manage even the busiest of days. "Even if you just take one breath before you pick up the calendar or the telephone or respond to the husband, you've made space for yourself!" Breathing techniques, mindfulness, contemplation, and other tools for journeying inward or tapping emotions will all serve to deepen your sense of inner peace. Like Helen, many women find that a journey of a thousand miles can begin with just one *breath*.

Building the body: Think of tending to your body as maintaining a temple. Exercise and good nutrition are akin to fortification. And they don't have to be a chore. Try to make exercise fun and meals mindful. Mindful eating can offer great enjoyment. So can a mindful walk or a yoga session. The best prescription for exercise involves choosing something you will *do*. Exercising for at least thirty minutes a day, most days of the week is ideal. But something is better than nothing. When you eat, be mindful, and work to include more nutritious foods (vegetables, whole grains, fruits, and calcium sources) into your diet.

Coping and Communication

You may think to yourself, if I had more time and fewer demands, doing all the "right things" would be easy. Stress is a major saboteur of the best-laid plans. However, since most of us can't leave for a deserted island anytime soon, we see no point in telling you to avoid stress entirely. The coping strategies we've discussed fall into two broad categories. Effective coping is a balance of both emotion- and problem-focused coping skills.

Research shows that optimistic (stress-hardy) people use prob-

Emotion-focused:	Problem-focused:
Relaxation response (RR)	*Direct action by changing:*
Monitoring thoughts	• Our communication style
Reframing	• An environment
Social support	• A schedule
Empathy	• A responsibility
Humor	• A family or work custom
Journal writing	• A procedure
Affirmations	• Our health habits
Contemplation	
Catharsis/venting:	
a good cry or laugh	

lem-focused coping much more readily than pessimists do, and that it tends to *keep* them optimistic. If you can solve a problem with direct action, do it. For example, if you want to get in shape, fix the plumbing, apologize to a friend, or lighten your load at work, problem-focused coping (direct action) is likely your best choice.

Emotion-focused coping also plays a critical role. We rely on emotion-focused coping to deflect stress and tap inner emotions. Teresa, who was having frequent arguments with her daughter, found that a daily practice of eliciting the RR and journaling (both emotion-focused coping skills) were helpful in decreasing feelings of anger. Teresa also went about setting boundaries, being more assertive

Mind Over Menopause Reminders

1. Elicit the relaxation response at least once per day.
2. Do "minis" as often as possible.
3. Practice "news and goods" on a daily basis.
4. Exercise regularly.
5. Do something nice for yourself as often as possible. Shoot for once a day.
6. Monitor what you eat.
7. Be mindful of each moment: eating, walking, cooking, cleaning, making love, driving. Learn to live in the here and now, not yesterday or tomorrow.
8. Monitor automatic negative thoughts. When you become aware of being anxious or upset, stop yourself, face the thought, and decide if it really is true.
9. Learn to recognize when you are anxious; be aware of how emotions reflect themselves in your body.
10. If you feel nagged by a disturbing event or conversation, write down that experience. Consider journaling.
11. Practice skills of effective communication. Really listen when someone talks to you; give them your undivided attention. Try to keep in mind the differences between assertive and aggressive communication. Assert yourself.
12. Recognize humor in your daily life.

Mind/Body Pearls of Wisdom

You cannot control the external circumstances of your life, but you can control your reactions to them.

In trying circumstances, reframe the situation as a challenge rather than a threat. In this way you acknowledge and nourish your own inner strength, even as you face doubt and uncertainty.

Change is the only constant in life.

If you have commitment, change is received with curiosity and openness, rather than with fear and doubt. If you feel resistant to change, try letting go and looking within. Seek answers in a contemplative meditation. Change can herald unexpected gains: self-expression, creativity, self-worth, and autonomy.

Accept yourself as you are.

Acceptance means actually honoring yourself as you are now. To the extent that you can honor your inner self, which—unlike your body—never changes, you become free from your own judgmental, negative thoughts. Keep a gratitude log nightly and practice affirmations throughout the day.

Live and let go.

The more accepting you become of yourself, the more you will see others in the same light. Forgive and see people for who they are instead of who you want them to be.

about her needs, and opening the lines of communication with her daughter (problem-focused coping). Using a combination of coping skills, both mother and daughter have gotten past the rocky times and now enjoy a good relationship.

Stay open to life's teachings.

There is an old aphorism that when the student is ready, the teacher will appear. The teacher may not be easily recognized. Sometimes the most difficult people are our greatest teachers of patience, forgiveness, and self-respect.

Journey inward.

Practice skills to make the journey inward. Listen to your inner wisdom and ask for what you need. Learn to trust your own judgment.

Breathe deeply.

Your breath is always with you, serving as the key to self-awareness and remembrance of your choices. In stressful circumstances, remember to breathe in and let your breath travel all the way out.

Go for the life you want.

Make more statements every day about what you want. Use the power of your meditation to create an image of what you want. Think grand, think positive, and . . . expect it to happen!

Boost Your Expectations

Your beliefs are incredibly powerful. So use them wisely. Imagine your life if you were to embody emotions of power, courage, compassion, or fulfillment on a daily basis. We say, try it! Some of the most powerful women in the world gain their crowning achievement after age fifty.

Gloria Steinem, Hillary Clinton, Jane Fonda, and Margaret Thatcher are among many women (some famous, others less well known) making the most of midlife. And you don't have to be a leader, an actress, or travel great distances to achieve success. There's much happiness to be found in any type of self-discovery. When asked if she felt closer to a higher power in space, Kathryn Sullivan, the first American woman to walk in space, observed, "I don't think hanging off the handrail of the spaceship in a space suit changes a person's core philosophy or values or spiritual views. Traveling two hundred miles anywhere doesn't put you farther or closer to anything. What I cherish is all the ways it stretched and taught and grew and educated and shaped and refined me." In many ways, Kathryn Sullivan had gained as much from the "journey" through learning and striving as she had from the "destination."

Sometimes our greatest accomplishment is the journey. Change is a journey and like any other trip, it's often filled with unexpected twists and turns, challenges that might cause you to take a few steps backward. There will be moments of frustration as well as elation. It is in the steps of change that we grow. Embrace the moments you love and negotiate the others. It is in learning, finding meaning, letting our truths surface, and embracing all that is around us that we reach our best. So, regardless of the path you choose, as the Nike ad says, "Just do it!"

The possibilities for all of us are endless as soon as we make the conscious decision to do things that will enrich us as human beings. Your Life Is Your Canvas, and remember, no one ever created great art by painting inside the lines.

—LORETTA LAROCHE

Glossary

androgens: Primarily male steroid hormones that are produced in the adrenal glands and ovaries in women.

antioxidant: A substance in food that helps to protect cells against damage from free radicals.

autonomic nervous system: The part of the nervous system that controls most of the body's automatic functions, such as temperature, heart rate, and blood pressure, through two parallel nerve systems, the sympathetic and the parasympathetic. It is also linked through the hypothalamus to the endocrine system.

body mass index (BMI): An estimate of an individual's relative body composition calculated from his or her height and weight.

central nervous system: Consists of the brain and the spinal cord. Receives sensory input and sends commands via the peripheral nervous system. Connects to the autonomic nervous system through the limbic system, particularly the hypothalamus.

cholesterol: A fat-like substance, produced by the liver and contained in all food from animal sources, that is an essential component of body cells and a precursor of bile acids and certain hormones.

chronic stress: A long-term, low-level hormonal reaction to continued stressors or perceived threats. In chronic stress, steroid hormones have negative effects on immunity, digestion, growth, and sexual function.

cognitive restructuring: Techniques intended to change the way people perceive or interpret an event, in order to reduce stress.

combined hormone therapy: Estrogen combined with progestin.

dual-energy X-ray absorptiometry (DXA): A test in which X rays limited to two different energies are used to measure bone density.

endometrium: The lining of the uterus.

epinephrine and norepinephrine: Also known as adrenaline and noradrenaline, they were the first stress-response hormones to be discovered. They kick off the

319

powerful fight-or-flight stress response. Epinephrine is secreted by the adrenal glands on top of the kidneys while norepinephrine is released by nerve endings of the sympathetic nervous system.

estradiol: Produced by the ovaries, the dominant form of estrogen in premenopausal women.

estrogen: A catchall term for primarily female steroid hormones that are produced in the ovaries, adrenal glands, placenta, and testes. In women, estrogen is responsible for the development of secondary sexual characteristics, the maturation and function of sexual organs, and the growth of the long bones.

estrogen therapy: Prescription estrogen therapy generally used to treat menopausal symptoms.

fatty acids: Constituents of fats; the essential fatty acids are those that the body cannot make on its own and therefore needs to obtain from dietary sources.

follicle stimulating hormone (FSH): A hormone secreted by the pituitary gland that stimulates the development of egg-containing follicles in the ovaries.

free radicals: A by-product of energy metabolism; these are highly reactive molecules that can damage cells, leaving them more vulnerable to other changes that can lead to heart disease and cancer.

glucocorticoids: The second class of hormones, after epinephrine, that is released by the adrenal glands during the stress response. The glucocorticoids are steroid hormones, affecting inflammation, blood pressure, and metabolism.

high-density lipoprotein (HDL): A "good" lipoprotein that protects the arteries by transporting cholesterol from body cells to the liver for elimination.

homocysteine: an amino acid that may be a risk factor for heart disease.

hormone therapy: Prescription estrogen and progestin therapies generally used to treat menopausal symptoms.

hot flash: A sudden feeling of heat in the face or upper part of the body, caused by the dilation of blood vessels in the skin and often accompanied by perspiration and flushing.

hydrogenation: The addition of hydrogen to a compound—particularly to unsaturated oils or soft fats—to harden them.

hypothalamus: The "master gland," the hypothalamus controls the dual nerve networks of the autonomic nervous system and, through the pituitary gland, the endocrine system.

hysterectomy: Surgical removal of the uterus.

immune system: The collective name for cells, chemicals, and physical barriers that defend the body against infections and protect against disease, including heart disease.

insulin: An anabolic (growth-promoting) hormone produced by the pancreas; it helps to metabolize glucose, amino acids, and fatty acids and store them in cells.

insulin resistance: A reduced sensitivity to insulin's action, which can contribute to type 2 diabetes.

limbic system: Located under the cerebral cortex, the limbic system consists of a number of key nerve centers, including the thalamus, hypothalamus, hippocampus, and amygdala, which are central to emotion, memory, and learning.

lipids: Fats, oils, and waxes that serve as building blocks for cells or as energy sources for the body.

lipoproteins: Protein-covered fat particles that enable cholesterol and trigylceride to move easily through the blood. The two main types of lipoprotein are high-density and low-density.

low-density lipoprotein (LDL): A "bad" lipoprotein that transports cholesterol from the liver to the rest of the body and can cause buildup of plaques in the arteries.

menopause: The point marking the end of menstruation and childbearing; defined by the World Health Organization as one year after the last period.

osteoporosis: A bone-thinning condition that can result in bone fracture.

perimenopause: Starting when periods become irregular and lasting until a year after menopause.

peripheral nervous system: The network of neurons that extends from the central nervous system to all other parts of the body, conveying signals and sensory information to and from the central nervous system.

placebo: An inert substance or treatment that has no active effect, given to patients in medical studies for comparison against a treatment that is expected to have active effects.

progesterone: A female steroid hormone, produced by the ovaries, that prepares the uterine lining for pregnancy.

progestin: A synthetic compound that produces effects similar to those of progesterone.

selective estrogen receptor modulator (SERM): A chemically synthesized drug that mimics estrogen in some tissues but acts to block estrogen's effects in others.

stress response: A short-term, intense hormonal reaction to a stressor. In what is sometimes called the fight-or-flight response, the brain signals through the hypothalamus to the endocrine system to release a cascade of chemical signals that prepare the body for emergency physical activity.

unopposed estrogen: Estrogen taken without a progestogen.

Organizations and Resources

Note: many of the following organizations provide helpful and convenient resource materials if requested. Each organization continually updates its listings, so inquiry is helpful in gathering the most up-to-date information.

American Association of Sex
Educators, Counselors and
Therapists (AASECT)
PO Box 5488
Richmond, VA 23220-0488
www.aasect.org

American Dietetic Association
216 Jackson Boulevard
Chicago, IL 60606-6995
(312) 899-0040
www.eatright.org

American Heart Association
7272 Greenville Avenue
Dallas, TX 75231
(214) 373-6300
www.americanheart.org

Center for Mindfulness in Medicine,
Health Care, and Society
University of Massachusetts Medical
School
55 Lake Avenue N.
Worcester, MA 01655
(508) 856-2656

www.umassmed.edu/cfm
www.mindfulnesstapes.com

Health Finder
www.healthfinder.gov

Massachusetts General Hospital
Center for Women's Mental Health
55 Fruit Street
Boston, MA 02114
(617) 726-2000
www.womensmentalhealth.org

Mind/Body Medical Institute
110 Francis Street
Boston, MA 02115
(617) 632-9543
www.mbmi.org

The Mind/Body Medical Institute offers a variety of audiotapes, videotapes, and CDs to help elicit the relaxation response and learn more about mind/body medicine. These can be ordered through the website or by calling the Mind/Body Medical Institute.

National Cancer Institute
Building 31, Room 10A03
31 Center Drive
Bethesda, MD 20892
(800) 4-CANCER
www.nci.nih.gov

National Center for Complementary
and Alternative Medicine, NIH
NCCAM Clearinghouse
P.O. Box 8218
Silver Spring, MD 20907-8218
(888) 644-6226
www.nccam.nih.gov

National Health Information Center
P.O. Box 1133
Washington, DC 20013-1133
(800) 336-4797
www.health.gov/nhic

National Heart Lung and Blood
Institute
P.O. Box 30105
Bethesda, MD 20824
(301) 592-8573
www.nhlbi.nih.gov

National Institute on Aging (NIA)
Building 31, Room 5C27
31 Center Drive, MSC 2292
Bethesda, MD 20892
(301) 496-1752
www.nih.gov/nia/
www.maillist.org/exercise

(Request: *Exercise: A Video from the
National Institute on Aging* and com-
panion booklet, $7.00)

National Institutes of Health
Bethesda, MD, 20892

(301) 496-4000
www.nih.gov
www.nih.gov/health/infoline.htm

National Institutes of Health
Osteoporosis and Related Bone
Diseases—National Resource
Center
1232 22nd Street NW
Washington, DC 20037
(800) 624-2663
www.osteo.org

(Request: *Boning Up on Osteoporosis: A Guide to Prevention and Treatment*)

National Osteoporosis Foundation
1232 22nd Street NW
Washington, DC 20037
(202) 223-2226
www.nof.org

(Request a free copy of: *The Role of
Exercise in the Prevention and Treatment of Osteoporosis*)

National PMS Society
P.O. Box 11467
Durham, NC 27703
(919) 489-6577

National Sleep Foundation
1522 K Street NW, Suite 500
Washington, DC 20005
(202) 347-3471
www.sleepfoundation.org

(Request: *Women and Sleep*)

National Women's Health Information
Center
(800) 994-9662 (800-994-WOMAN)
www.4women.gov

North American Menopause Society
P.O. Box 94527
Cleveland, OH 44101
(800) 774-5342
www.menopause.org

(Request: *The Menopause Guidebook*)

Sexual Health Network
www.sexualhealth.com

NEWSLETTERS

A Friend Indeed
Box 260
Pembina, ND 58271
(294) 989-8028
www.afriendindeed.ca

Harvard Women's Health Watch
Harvard Health Publications
10 Shattuck Street, Suite 612
Boston, MA 02115
www.health.harvard.edu

HerbalGram
American Botanical Council
6200 Manor Road
Austin, TX 78723
(800) 373-7105
www.herbalgram.org

(Offers a quarterly magazine)

The Soy Connection
Communique, Inc.
P.O. Box 237
Jefferson City, MO 65102
(573) 635-3265
www.talksoy.com

*Tufts University Health & Nutrition
Letter: Your Guide to Living
Healthier Longer*
Tufts University
P.O. Box 420235
Palm Coast, FL 32142
(800) 274-7581
www.healthletter.tufts.edu

ADDITIONAL RESOURCES

Soy Products

These websites offer information on
healthy eating, as well as a wide range
of soy products and a variety of recipes.

www.dixiediner.com
www.nasoya.com
www.kashi.com
www.morningstarfarms.com
www.bocaburger.com

Exercise/Yoga Videos

Try visiting these websites to find out
more about exercise and yoga and how
each can help you keep feeling healthy
and grounded.

GENERAL

www.Strongwomen.com
www.jane-fonda.net

YOGA

www.kripalu.com (Video: *Kripalu Yoga: Gentle with Carolyn Lundeen Sudha*)

www.yogaheart.com (800) 558-YOGA (Video: *Embracing Menopause: A Path to Peace and Power*)

Sexual Exploration

Sexuality can sometimes be an awkward topic to broach with your clinician or even a partner. These websites offer various products for women who may want to add something different to their sex lives.

www.evesgarden.com

www.grandopening.com

Learning to Laugh

A sense of humor can come in handy when dealing with the added stress of going through menopause. These websites offer articles, videotapes, books, and even e-cards for those women looking for an excuse to smile.

www.mbmi.org

www.stressed.com

www.thelaughoutloudcompany.com

Selected Books

MENOPAUSE AND WOMEN'S HEALTH

Note: The North American Menopause Society publishes "Menopause and Beyond: Suggested Reading for Informed Decision-Making." This is an excellent guide to good literature on the subject. We also suggest the following:

Barbach, Lonnie. *The Pause: Positive Approaches to Perimenopause and Menopause* (2nd ed.). New York: The Penguin Group, 2000.

Berman, Jennifer, Laura Berman, and Elisabeth Bunmiller. *For Women Only: A Revolutionary Guide to Overcoming Sexual Dysfunction and Reclaiming Your Sex Life*. New York: Henry Holt, 2001.

Borysenko, Joan. *A Woman's Book of Life*. New York: Riverhead Books, 1996.

The Boston Women's Health Book Collective. *Our Bodies, Ourselves for the New Century: A Book by and for Women*. New York: Simon & Schuster, 1998.

DeAngelo, Debbie. *Sudden Menopause: Restoring Health & Emotional Well-Being*. Alameda, CA: Hunter House Publishers, 2001.

Gaston, Marilyn, and Gayle Porter. *Prime Time: The African American Woman's Complete Guide to Midlife Health and Wellness*. New York: Ballantine Publishing Group, 2001.

Greenwood, Sadja. *Menopause, Naturally: Preparing for the Second Half of Life*. Volcano, CA: Volcano Press, 1996.

Hankinson, Susan E., R.N., Sc.D.; Colditz, Graham A., M.D.; Manson, JoAnn, M.D.; and Speizer, Frank E., M.D. *Healthy Women, Healthy Lives: A Guide to Preventing Disease*. New York: Simon & Schuster, 2001.

Hudson, Tori. *Women's Encyclopedia of Natural Medicine: Alternative Therapies and Integrative Medicine*. Los Angeles: Keats Publishing, 1999.

Love, Susan. *Dr. Susan Love's Breast Book* (3rd ed.). Cambridge, MA: Perseus Publishing, 2000.

Love, Susan. *Dr. Susan Love's Hormone Book*. New York: Random House, 1997.

Lynch, Lee, and Akia Woods, eds. *Off the Rag: Lesbians Writing on Menopause.* Norwich, VT: New Victoria Publishers, 1996.

Sichel, Deborah, and Jeanne Driscoll. *Women's Moods: What Every Woman Must Know about Hormones, the Brain, and Emotional Health.* New York: William Morrow, 1999.

National Women's Health Network. *The Truth About Hormone Replacement Therapy: How to Break Free from the Medical Myths of Menopause.* New York: Prima Lifestyles, 2002.

Voda, Ann, R.N., Ph.D. *Menopause, Me and You.* Binghamton, NY: Haworth Press, 1997.

MIND/BODY

Mind/Body Medical Institute Affiliated Books

Benson, Herbert. *Beyond the Relaxation Response: How to Harness the Healing Power of Your Personal Beliefs.* New York: Times Books, 1984.

Benson, Herbert. *The Breakout Principle.* New York: Scribner, 2003.

Benson, Herbert. *The Relaxation Response.* New York: Avon Books, 1975.

Benson, Herbert. *Timeless Healing: The Power and Biology of Belief.* New York: Scribner, 1996.

Benson, Herbert, and Eileen Stuart. *The Wellness Book: The Comprehensive Guide to Treating Stress-Related Illness.* New York: Carol Publishing Group, 1992.

Domar, Alice D., and Henry Dreher. *Healing Mind, Healthy Woman: Using the Mind-Body Connection to Manage Stress and Take Control of Your Life.* New York: Bantam Doubleday, 1997.

Domar, Alice D., and Henry Dreher. *Self-Nurture: Learning to Care for Yourself as Effectively as You Care for Everyone Else.* New York: Viking Penguin, 1999.

Jacobs, Gregg D. *The Ancestral Mind: Reclaim the Power.* New York: Viking Press, 2003.

Jacobs, Gregg D. *Say Good Night to Insomnia.* New York: Henry Holt, 1998.

Additional Books

Borysenko, Joan. *Minding the Body, Mending the Mind.* New York: Bantam, 1993.

Burns, David. *Feeling Good: The New Mood Therapy.* New York: William Morrow, 1980.

Burns, David. *The Feeling Good Handbook, Revised.* New York: Plume, 1999.

Cameron, Julia. *The Artist's Way.* New York: Penguin Putnam, 1992.

Das, Lama Surya. *Awakening the Buddha Within.* New York: Broadway Books, 1998.

Fontana, David. *Learn to Meditate: A Practical Guide to Self-Discovery and Fulfillment*. San Francisco: Chronicle Books, 1999.

Frankl, Viktor E. *Man's Search for Meaning*. New York: Washington Square Press, 1997.

Grabhorn, Lynn. *Excuse Me, Your Life Is Waiting*. Charlottesville, VA: Hampton Roads, 2000.

Jeffers, Susan. *Feel the Fear and Do It Anyway*. New York: Harcourt, 1990.

Kabat-Zinn, Jon. *Full Catastrophic Living*. New York: Delacourt, 1990.

Kabat-Zinn, Jon. *Wherever You Go, There You Are: Mindfulness Meditation in Everyday Life*. New York: Hyperion, 1994.

Khan, Pir Vilayat Inayat. *Awakening: A Sufi Experience*. New York: Tarcher, 1999.

Langer, Ellen J. *Mindfulness* (7th ed.). Reading, MA: Addison-Wesley, 1994.

Lerner, Harriet. *The Dance of Anger: A Woman's Guide to Changing the Patterns of Intimate Relationships*. New York: Harper and Row, 1985.

Levine, Stephen. *Guided Meditations, Explorations and Healings*. New York: Anchor Books, Doubleday, 1991.

McEwen, Bruce. *The End of Stress As We Know It*. Washington DC: National Academics Press, 2002.

Nhat Hanh, Thich. *The Miracle of Mindfulness: An Introduction to the Practice of Meditation*. Boston: Beacon Press, 1999.

Rowe, John W., and Robert L. Kahn. *Successful Aging*. New York: Dell Publishing, 1998.

Seligman, Martin. *Authentic Happiness*. New York: Free Press, 2002.

Seligman, Martin. *Learned Optimism*. New York: Simon & Schuster, 1998.

Williams, Redford, and Virginia Williams. *Anger Kills: Seventeen Strategies for Controlling the Hostility that Can Harm Your Health*. New York: Harper Mass Market Paperback, 1998.

Williams, Redford, and Virginia Williams. *Lifeskills: Eight Simple Ways to Build Stronger Relationships, Communicate More Clearly, and Improve Health*. New York: Times Books, 1999.

Yoga and Exercise

American College of Sports Medicine. *ACSM Fitness Book* (3rd ed.). Human Kinetics, 2003.

Anderson, Sandra, and Rolf Sovic. *Yoga: Mastering the Basics*. Homedale, PA: Himalayan Institute Press, 2002.

Francina, Suza. *The New Yoga for People Over 50*. Deerfield Beach, FL: Health Communications, 1977.

Francina, Suza. *Yoga and the Wisdom of Menopause*. Deerfield Beach, FL: Health Communications, 2003.

Lasater, Judith. *Relax and Renew: Restful Yoga for Stressful Times.* Berkeley, CA: Rodmell Press, 1995.

Lynch, Jerry, and Al Chungliang Huang. *Working Out, Working Within: The Tao on Inner Fitness Through Sports.* New York: Jeremy P. Tarcher/Putnam, 1998.

Maddern, Jan. *Yoga Builds Bones: Easy Gentle Stretches that Prevent Osteoporosis.* Boston: Element, 2000.

Manson, JoAnn, and Patricia Amend. *The 30-Minute Fitness Solution: A Four-Step Plan for Women of All Ages.* Cambridge, MA: Harvard University Press, 2001.

Nelson, Miriam. *Strong Women Stay Young.* New York: Bantam Books, 2000.

Nelson, Miriam. *Strong Women, Strong Bones,* New York: G.P. Putnam's Sons, 2000.

Scott Kortge, Carolyn. *The Spirited Walker: Fitness Walking for Clarity, Balance, and Spiritual Connection.* San Francisco: Harper San Francisco, 1998.

Diet and Nutrition

Beck, Leslie. *Managing Menopause with Diet and Herbs: An Essential Guide for the Peri and Post Menopausal Years.* Toronto: Prentice Hall Canada, 2000.

Bronfman, David and Rachelle. *CalciYum! Delicious Calcium-Rich, Dairy-Free Vegetarian Recipes.* Toronto: Bromedia, 1998.

Fletcher, Anne, and Jane Brody. *Thin for Life: Ten Keys to Success from People Who Have Lost Weight and Kept It Off.* New York: Houghton Mifflin, 2001.

Heber, D. *What Color Is Your Diet?* New York: Harper Collins, 2001.

Reaven, G. M., T. K. Strom, and B. Fox. *Syndrome X, The Silent Killer: The New Heart Disease Risk.* New York: Fireside, 2001.

Shandler, Nina. *Estrogen the Natural Way: Over 250 Easy and Delicious Recipes for Menopause.* New York: Villard Books, 1997.

Waterhouse, Debra. *Outsmarting the Midlife Fat Cell: Winning Weight Control Strategies for Women over 35 to Stay Fit through Menopause.* New York: Hyperion, 1999.

Willett, Walter C. *Eat, Drink, and Be Healthy: The Harvard Medical School Guide to Healthy Eating.* New York: Simon & Schuster, 2001.

Selected Sources by Chapter

CHAPTER 1. REDEFINING "THE CHANGE"

Benson, Herbert, and Eileen Stuart. *The Wellness Book: The Comprehensive Guide to Maintaining Health and Treating Stress-Related Illness*. New York: Carol Publishing Group, 1992.

Koenig, Harold, M.D. "The Effects of Stress, Relaxation, and Belief on Health and Healthcare Costs," *Testimony to the United States Senate Appropriations Subcommittee on Labor/HHS & Education*, September 22, 1998.

North American Menopause Society. *Menopause Core Curriculum Study Guide*, 2002. Update consumer guides available from http://www.menopause.org.

CHAPTER 2. UNDERSTANDING HORMONAL CHANGES

Hot flashes/ general

Kronenberg, F. "Hot Flashes." In R.A. Lobo, ed., *Treatment of the Postmenopausal Woman: Basic and Clinical Aspects* (2nd ed.). Philadelphia: Lippincott Williams & Wilkins, 1999.

Kronenberg, F. "Hot Flashes: Phenomenology, Quality of Life, and Search for Treatment Options." *Experimental Gerontology* 29/3–4 (1994): 319–336.

Insomnia

Jacobs, Gregg D. *Say Good Night to Insomnia*. New York: Henry Holt, 1998.

Owens, J.F., and Matthews, K.A. "Sleep Disturbance in Healthy Middle-aged Women," *Maturitas* 30/1 (September 20, 1998): 41–50.

Shaver, Joan L.F., Shannon N. Zenk, et al. "Sleep Disturbances in Menopause," *Journal of Women's Health & Gender-based Medicine* 9/2 (November 2, 2000): 109–118.

Mood/PMS

Avis, N.E., S. Crawford, R. Stellato, and C. Longcope. "Longitudinal Study of Hormone Levels and Depression Among Women Transitioning Through Menopause." *Climacteric* 4/3 (2001): 243–249.

Goodale, I.L., Domar, A.D., and Benson, H. "Alleviation of Premenstrual Syndrome Symptoms with the Relaxation Response," *Obstetrics and Gynecology* 75/4 (April 1990): 649–655.

Woods, N.F., et al. "Patterns of Depressed Mood Across the Menopausal Transition: Approaches to Studying Patterns in Longitudinal Data." *Acta Obstetrica et Gynecologica Scandinavica* 81 (2002): 623–632.

Woods, N.F., and E.S. Mitchell. "Pathways to Depressed Mood for Midlife Women: Observations from the Seattle Midlife Women's Health Study." *Research in Nursing and Health* 2 (April 20, 1997): 119–129.

Memory

Komaroff, A.L., ed. *Improving Your Memory, A Special Report from Harvard Medical School*. Boston: Harvard Health Publications, 2002.

Woods, N.F., Mitchell, E.S., and Adams, C. "Memory Functioning Among Midlife women, Observations from the Seattle Midlife Women's Health Study." *Menopause* 7/4 (2000): 257–265.

Sexuality

Avis, N.E., et al. "Is There an Association Between Menopause Status and Sexual Functioning?" *Menopause: The Journal of The North American Menopause Society* 7/5 (September–October 2000): 297–309.

Avis, N.E., et al. "Sexual Function and Aging in Men and Women: Community and Population Based Studies." *Gender Specific Medicine* 3/2 (March–April 2000): 37–41.

Butler, R.N. "Love and Sex after 60" [Editorial]. *Geriatrics* 49/9 (September 1994): 10–11.

Butler, R.N., et al. "Love and Sex after 60: How Physical Changes Affect Intimate Expression. A Roundtable Discussion: Part 1." *Geriatrics* 49/9 (September 1994): 20–27.

Dennerstein, L., et al. "Factors Affecting Sexual Functioning of Women in the Mid-Life Years." *Climacteric* 2/4 (December 1999): 254–262.

Dennerstein, L., et al. "Hormones, Mood, Sexuality, and the Menopausal Transition." *Fertility and Sterility* 77/4, Suppl. 4 (April 2002): 42–48.

Jacoby, S. "Great Sex: What's Age Got to Do with It?" (summary of AARP/*Modern*

Maturity Sexuality Survey findings). *Modern Maturity* (September–October 1999): 43–48.

Osteoporosis

Michelson, D., et al. "Bone Mineral Density in Women with Depression." *New England Journal of Medicine* 335 (October 17, 1996): 1176–1181.
Nelson, Miriam. *Strong Women, Strong Bones.* New York: G.P. Putnam's Sons, 2000.

Heart Disease

American Heart Association. *2001 Heart and Stroke Statistical Update.* Dallas, TX: American Heart Association, 2000.

CHAPTER 3. THE RELAXATION RESPONSE

Benson, H. *The Relaxation Response.* New York: Avon Books, 1975.
Benson, H. *Timeless Healing.* New York: Scribner, 1996.
Chrousos, George, et al. "The Concepts of Stress and Stress System Disorders; Overview of Physical and Behavioral Homeostasis." *Journal of the American Medical Association* 267/9 (March 4, 1992): 1244–1252.
Ferrin, M. "Stress and the Reproductive Cycle." *Journal of Clinical Endocrinology & Metabolism* 84/6 (1999): 1768–1774.
Hoffman, J.W., et al. "Reduced Sympathetic Nervous System Responsivity Associated with the Relaxation Response." *Science* 215 (1982): 190–192.

CHAPTER 4. SELF-NURTURE

Covey, Stephen. *The 7 Habits of Highly Effective People: Powerful Lessons in Personal Change.* New York: A Fireside Book, 1989.
Domar, Alice D., and Henry Dreher. *Healing Mind, Healthy Woman.* New York: Bantam Doubleday, 1996.
Domar, Alice D., and Henry Dreher. *Self-Nurture.* New York: Viking Penguin, 2000.

CHAPTER 5. EXERCISE: MOVING THROUGH MENOPAUSE

Blumenthal, J.A., et al. "Exercise Treatment for Major Depression: Maintenance of Therapeutic Benefit at 10 Months." *Psychosomatic Medicine* 62 (2000): 633–638.

Huddleston, J.S. "Exercise," in Edelman, C., and C. Mandle, eds., *Health Promotion Throughout the Lifespan* (5th ed.). St. Louis, MO: Mosby-Year Book, 2002.

Manson, J., et al. "A Prospective Study of Walking as Compared with Vigorous Exercise in the Prevention of Coronary Heart Disease in Women." *New England Journal of Medicine* 341 (1999): 650–658.

National Institutes of Health Consensus Development Panel on Physical Activity and Cardiovascular Health. "Physical Activity and Cardiovascular Health." *Journal of the American Medical Association* 276 (1996): 241–246.

Pate, R.R., et al. "Physical Activity and Public Health: A Recommendation from the Centers for Disease Control and Prevention and the American College of Sports Medicine." *Journal of the American Medical Association* 273 (1995): 402–407.

U.S. Department of Health and Human Services. *Physical Activity Fundamental to Preventing Disease,* June 20, 2002. aspe.hhs.gov/health/reports/physical activity/physicalactivity.pdf

Williford, H.N., et al. "Exercise Prescription for Women." *Sports Medicine* 15 (1993): 299–311.

Wolff, I., J.J. van Croonenborg, H.C. Kemper, P.J. Kostenese, and J.W. Twisk. "The Effect of Exercise Training Programs on Bone Mass: A Meta-Analysis of Published Controlled Trials in Pre- and Postmenopausal Women." *Osteoporosis Int.* 9/1 (1999): 1–12.

CHAPTER 6. NUTRITION:
THE HEALING PLATE

Anderson, J.W., B.M. Johnstone, and M.E. Cook-Newell. "Meta-Analysis of the Effects of Soy Protein Intake on Serum Lipids." *New England Journal of Medicine* 333 (1995): 276–282.

Hodish, I., et al. "Effect of Elevated Homocysteine Levels on Clinical Restenosis Following Percutaneous Coronary Intervention." *Cardiology* 97 (2002): 214–217.

Hu, F.B., et al. "Fish and Omega-3 Fatty Acid Intake and Risk of Coronary Heart Disease in Women." *Journal of the American Medical Association* 287 (2002): 1815–1821.

National Heart, Lung, and Blood Institute. *Third Report of the National Cholesterol Education Program Expert Panel on Detection, Evaluation, and Treatment of High Blood Cholesterol in Adults.* Bethesda, MD: National Institutes of Health, May 2001.

Willett, W.C., ed. *Eat, Drink and Be Healthy: The Harvard Medical School Guide to Healthy Eating.* New York: Simon & Schuster, 2001.

CHAPTER 7. POSTMENOPAUSAL HORMONE THERAPY

Grady, D., et al. HERS Research Group. "Cardiovascular Disease Outcomes During 6.8 Years of Hormone Therapy: Heart and Estrogen/Progestin Replacement Study Follow-up (HERS II)." *Journal of the American Medical Association* 288/1 (July 3, 2002): 49–57.

Hulley, S., et al. HERS Research Group. "Noncardiovascular Disease Outcomes During 6.8 Years of Hormone Therapy: Heart and Estrogen/Progestin Replacement Study Follow-up (HERS II)." *Journal of the American Medical Association* 288/1 (July 3, 2002): 58–64.

National Institutes of Health, menopausal hormone therapy information. http://www.nih.gov/PHTindex.htm

Nurses' Health Study. http://www.channing.harvard.edu/nhs/

Petitti, D.B. "Hormone Replacement Therapy for Prevention: More Evidence, More Pessimism." Editorial, *Journal of the American Medical Association* 288/1 (July 3, 2002): 99–101.

CHAPTER 8. MANAGING SYMPTOMS

Butler, R.N., et al. "Love and Sex after 60: How to Evaluate and Treat the Sexually Active Woman." A Roundtable Discussion: Part 3. *Geriatrics* 49/11 (November 1994): 33–4, 37–8, 41–2.

Freedman, R.R. "Hot Flash Etiology: New Directions for Research." *Menopause Management* 11/4 (July/August 2002): 8.

Freedman, R.R. "Hot Flash Trends and Mechanisms" (editorial). *Menopause* 9/3 (2002): 151–152.

Freedman, R.R., and S. Woodward. "Behavioral Treatment of Menopausal Hot Flushes: Evaluation by Ambulatory Monitoring." *American Journal of Obstetrics & Gynecology* 167/2 (1992): 436–439.

Irvin, J.H., A.D. Domar, et al. "The Effects of Relaxation Response Training on Menopausal Symptoms." *Journal of Psychosomatic Obstetrics and Gynecology* 17 (1996): 202–207.

Kronenberg, Fredi, Adriane Fugh-Berman, et al. "Complementary and Alternative Medicine for Menopausal Symptoms: A Review of Randomized, Controlled Trials." *Annals of Internal Medicine* 137 (2002): 805–813. Available from http://www.annals.org.

Loprinzi, Charles L., et al. "Venlafaxine in Management of Hot Flashes in Survivors of Breast Cancer: A Randomised Controlled Trial." *Lancet* 356 (2000): 2059–63.

North American Menopause Society. *Menopause Core Curriculum Guide*, 2002. Updated consumer guides available from http://www.menopause.org.

Sarrel, P.M., and M.I. Whitehead. "Sex and Menopause: Defining the Issues." *Maturitas* 7/3 (September 1985): 217–24.

Shaver, J.L.F. "Beyond Hormonal Therapies in Menopause." *Experimental Gerontology* 29/3–4 (1994): 469–476.

CHAPTER 9. PROTECTING YOUR HEALTH

Kaufmann, M.W., et al. "Relation Between Myocardial Infarction, Depression, Hostility and Death." *American Heart Journal* 138 (1999): 549–554.

Komaroff, A.L., Editor in Chief. *A Guide to Alzheimer's Disease, A Special Report from Harvard Medical School.* Boston: Harvard Health Publications, 2002.

North American Menopause Society. *Report from the NAMS Advisory Panel on Postmenopausal Hormone Therapy,* October 3, 2002. Available from http://www.menopause.org.

Women's Health Initiative. "New Facts About: Estrogen/Progestin Hormone Therapy." Available from http://www.whi.org.

CHAPTER 10. THE POWER OF YOUR MIND

Avis, N.E. and S.M. McKinlay. "A Longitudinal Analysis of Women's Attitudes Toward the Menopause: Results from the Mass Women's Health Study." *Maturitas* 13/1 (March 1991): 65–79.

Burns, D. *Feeling Good: The New Mood Therapy.* New York: William Morrow, 1980; repr. Avon Books, 1999.

Ellis, A., and R. Grieger. *Handbook of Rational-Emotive Therapy, Volume II.* New York: Springer, 1986.

LaRoche, Loretta. *Relax—You May Only Have a Few Minutes Left.* New York: Villard Books, 1998.

Lock, M. "The Contested Meanings of the Menopause." *Lancet* 337 (May 25, 1991): 1270.

Smith, Huston. *The Illustrated World's Religions: A Guide to Our Wisdom Traditions.* San Francisco: HarperCollins, 1995.

CHAPTER 11. RESILIENCY: INNER STRENGTH

LaRoche, Loretta. *Life Is Not a Stress Rehearsal.* New York: Broadway Books, 2001.

Lerner, Harriet. *The Dance of Anger: A Woman's Guide to Changing the Patterns of Intimate Relationships* New York: Harper and Row, 1985.

Maddi, S., and S. Kobasa. *The Hardy Executive: Health Under Stress.* Chicago: Dorsey Professional Books, 1984.

Pennebaker, J.W. "Writing Your Wrongs." *American Health,* January/February 1991, pp. 64–67. Adapted from Pennebaker, J.W., *Opening Up: The Healing Power of Confiding in Others.* New York: William Morrow, 1990.

Pennebaker, J.W., and J.D. Seagal. "Forming a Story: The Health Benefits of Narrative." *Journal of Clinical Psychology* 55 (1999): 1243–1254.

ILLUSTRATION CREDITS

Unless otherwise noted, all art and tables are provided courtesy of the Mind/Body Medical Institute and Harvard Health Publications.

Unless otherwise noted, all visualization exercises are provided by the Mind/Body Medical Institute.

Three Legged Stool illustrated by Amy Yeager.

Hormone Production in Women illustrated by Scott Leighton.

The Hormonal Dance drawing adapted by Scott Leighton from R. Barbieri, A. Domar, and K. Loughlin, *Six Steps to Increased Fertility* (New York: Simon & Schuster, 2000).

Savasana reprinted by permission of the artist, David Sipress.

Sample Time Pie from A. Domar and H. Dreher, *Self-Nurture* (New York: Viking Penguin, 2000).

Perceived Exertion illustrated by Jim Huddleston, adapted from "Borg Scale of Perceived Exertion" in G. A. Borg, "Psychophysical Basis of Perceived Exertion," *Medicine and Science in Sports and Exercise* 14 (1982): 377.

How to Burn About 150 Calories from *Physical Activity and Health: A Report of the Surgeon General* (Washington, D.C.: U.S. Department of Health and Human Services, 1996).

The New Healthy Eating Pyramid adapted from Dr. Walter Willett, *Eat, Drink, and Be Healthy: The Harvard Medical School Guide to Healthy Eating* (New York: Simon & Schuster, 2001).

Challenging Cognitive Distortions adapted from David D. Burns, M.D., *Feeling Good: The New Mood Therapy* (New York: William Morrow, 1980; repr. Avon Books, 1999).

Index

About the Authors

LESLEE KAGAN, M.S., N.P., director of the Mind/Body Program for Menopause and codirector of the Mind/Body Program for Infertility since 1999, has twenty years of clinical experience as a nurse practitioner in the field of women's health. Her work in menopause has been recognized by the North American Menopause Society. She also trains other health care professionals throughout the United States in the application of mind/body medicine to women.

BRUCE KESSEL, M.D., is an associate professor in the Department of Obstetrics, Gynecology, and Women's Health at the University of Hawaii and a member of the board of trustees of the North American Menopause Society.

HERBERT BENSON, M.D., is the founding president of the Mind/Body Medical Institute and the Mind/Body Medical Institute Associate Professor of Medicine, Harvard Medical School. A pioneer in mind/body medicine, he defined the relaxation response and continues to lead teaching and research into its efficacy in counteracting the harmful effects of stress.